UNIVERSAL
COVERAGE

A NOVEL

UNIVERSAL COVERAGE

A NOVEL

DANIEL PUTKOWSKI

HAWSER

UNIVERSAL COVERAGE Copyright © 2009 by Daniel Putkowski
All rights reserved. Printed in the United States of America.

ISBN 978-0-9815959-4-8

FIRST HAWSER PRESS EDITION DECEMBER 2009
10 9 8 7 6 5 4 3 2 1

danielputkowski.com

SALVARE, YOUR HEALTHCARE ALTERNATIVE / :60 TELEVISION SPOT

PROLOGUE

VIDEO	AUDIO
(FADE IN) Salvare *at sea moving swiftly over the waves*	**(SFX)waves crashing (MUSIC)soothing (NARRATOR)female:** Afraid you might not receive critical treatment before it's too late? Consider a visit to *Salvare,* your healthcare alternative.
(CUT TO) *Patients standing in line at HAO, waiting to schedule appointments*	Perhaps you're waiting for open heart surgery or chemotherapy. Maybe you've been turned down for a knee or hip replacement. *Salvare* offers you the option of prompt service in these and many more medical specialties.
(CUT TO) Salvare *staff posed on deck, smiling*	Our doctors trained and practiced in institutions that were once household names. Now they bring their skills to *Salvare,* located in international waters off the coast of Cape May, New Jersey.
(MONTAGE) Salvare *exterior, private staterooms, dining facilities, helicopter landing on* Salvare, *patient consulting with doctor, patient enjoying pool and other amenities*	A 120,000 ton displacement ocean liner, *Salvare,* features private staterooms for every patient, chef-prepared meals, nightly entertainment, and plenty of space for your loved ones to join you.\n\nMore than a hospital, *Salvare* is an integrated medical services facility that takes your healthcare experience to a new level. From the moment you arrive via helicopter, to your consultation with our physicians, until your recovery is complete, you will find yourself in an environment where the needs of the patient come first.

VIDEO	AUDIO
(FADE IN) *Jossy standing on helipad on Salvare's bow, scroll website and toll-free number on ticker: THE-SALVARE.com*	**STEVEN JOSSY, M.D.:** Hello! I'm Dr. Steven Jossy, founder and director of *Salvare,* your healthcare alternative. Don't waste precious time waiting at your HAO trying to schedule another appointment. Call our toll-free number today and reserve a seat aboard the next flight to our wonderful ship. I personally greet you upon arrival and will check in to make sure your treatment is going according to plan. Call today. Timing is everything.
(FADE TO BLACK) *Scroll legal disclaimer text*	**NARRATOR(female):** The preceding message is a commercial advertisement and is not endorsed by the Universal Coverage System. The medical facility mentioned is neither licensed by the United States Government, nor staffed by personnel certified under the requirements set forth in the Universal Healthcare and Medical Assistance Act, including any amendments thereto. Visiting such a facility without prior approval from the Healthcare Administration Authority may result in the suspension of your Universal Coverage benefits, the assessment of a fine, and/or in the case of fraud, punishment up to but not exceeding one year in prison as determined by the Healthcare Administration Authority, Medical Service Bureau.

"ARE YOU A DOCTOR, MR. SMITH?"

CHAPTER ONE

BOB SMITH STOOD LESS THAN TEN FEET from the President of the United States. It was a heady thrill, being this close to the only chief executive for whom he'd voted. Although they made eye contact several times, he didn't dare introduce himself. Still, in those clipped moments, Smith felt as if he'd made a solid connection with the man, that he could step up, extend his hand and start chatting. He might mention that during his grad school years he'd been part of the campaign.

However, Smith was among the lesser dignitaries at the reception, a mere senior engineer employed by the host of the event, Mark Wexler, CEO of Wexler Associates. While there were a few other Wexler employees present, the rest of the honored guests held more significant titles such as governor, congressman, senator, and mayor. Then there were the union bosses and the owners of the construction firms. A few hardhats, men who actually operated machinery and got their hands dirty in the course of building something, hovered near the makeshift bar that had been set up in Wexler's largest conference room.

From the floor to ceiling windows, Smith searched the cityscape for the stage on which this same group had gathered only an hour earlier. They came to a barren site in the middle of a distressed neighborhood to hear the President speak. Everyone, including a crowd of several thousand, wanted to know just what they were due to receive from the federal stimulus package. The surprise was a long time coming because the President wanted to talk about his other plans first, and he wasn't shy about expounding upon them. He was known to ramble for an hour or more, frequently alternating between a lecture and a pep talk.

Today's message centered on a new educational initiative aimed at controlling the cost of college and graduate school. The hardhats managed to hide their obscene gestures at this point but just barely. Smith, on the other hand, welcomed the news that there would be government funding for higher education. He had an eleven-year-old son, Timmy, and had only just begun saving tuition money. Although it was too early to be sure, Smith believed Timmy had a chance at a baseball scholarship. A local Little League coach had recruited Timmy to play for the Media Moguls, saying that he hadn't seen natural talent like his in years.

Then, almost as an afterthought, the President announced that the time had finally come for the redevelopment of this blighted piece of Philadelphia. The crowd rewarded him with a round of applause, which was one part relief that his previous talk had ended and another part elation that a chunk of money was coming their way. The noise didn't end until he raised both hands in a plea for quiet. Stimulus funds had been approved for the construction of a brand new medical facility to be known as the Philadelphia Central West District Health Services and Community Support Center, or Central West for short. Naturally, this long suffering area needed associated commercial spaces: a shopping mall, multiplex cinema, and plenty of restaurants. Finally, there would be residential towers to increase the supply of affordable housing. All this would provide a handsome return on the taxpayers' investment in the future. More applause, hoots, and whistles confirmed the President's assertion.

Like so many others, Smith believed in this policy. After all, Wexler Associates had designed the project on spec and was lucky enough to be selected as the winning proposal, which meant his job was secure. As he rode back to the office, Smith envisioned the equipment that was already en route to the site. Soon the foundation would be in the ground. And now, from his vantage point in the conference room, while everyone else chatted and sipped drinks, he imagined the buildings that would stand above that foundation.

It would take three years to finish Central West, during which time Smith knew the economy would be back on its feet and more work would flood the offices of Wexler Associates. The President was a tireless cheerleader of the people. His contagious energy inspired young and old alike, which left Smith somewhere in the middle as he had long ago left college yet was too far from retirement to even mention the word.

He heard Mark Wexler calling his name, but Smith was transfixed by his view of the city. He simply couldn't look away from the future.

man on the foundation team.

"Elvis has left the building," Josh kidded, referring to the President.

"I have to go," Smith said. "My son's in the hospital."

"Go! Go! Wait, do you need any help?"

"No. Sorry Josh, you'll have to find a ride home."

"Forget it. Go! Call me with the good news when you have it."

With that Smith bolted through the doorway.

He drove like a fool, exceeding the speed limit and slowing down just enough to make it through red lights without waiting for them to change. Between thoughts of his son, Smith couldn't help but be grateful for the extra gasoline ration in his fuel tank. Without it, he would've had to stop for gas, typically half an hour's delay, maybe longer.

The upside of energy rationing was sparse traffic on both the interstate and local roads. Gripping the wheel, he nodded in affirmation that the government had done the right thing with the Federal Energy Management Program. When it really counted, as in the case of this situation with Timmy, the lanes were open for those who truly needed them instead of people simply driving about inefficiently, wasting gas, and causing traffic jams. As an engineer, Smith appreciated the elegance of central planning. Had it not been a case of his son's health, he would have smiled at the effectiveness of the program, which was one pushed hard by the President he had just met.

But his son was in the emergency room. There would be no smiling until the boy was the happy, smart, enthusiastic child Smith and Hannah raised to this point. He forgot about national planning, gasoline rationing, and open highways. For all he knew, his son's life was in danger. He wanted the details, and he wanted them immediately from a professional like himself, someone who knew what they were doing in their chosen field.

Not since his father had fallen off a roof many years ago had Smith been to an emergency room. He was shocked by the condition of the facility at Media General, a hospital built to consolidate other smaller ones in the area. It offended his sense of competent order. An unruly gaggle of people loitered on rows of plastic benches, which were flanked by overflowing trashcans. The rough carpet had been worn through in places and pocked by hideous stains. And the noise, it was nearly deafening. People shouted across the room at a blaring television set. A woman with a clipboard hollered names. Giggling children, one with a bleeding ear, chased each other through the obstacle course formed by the seats.

Smith elbowed his way through a knot of people blocking the reception window. He struck one man particularly hard, and for a moment, thought the guy might retaliate. Just then an opening appeared between two bawling women. Smith threaded through them and made it to the window unmolested.

An empty desk on the other side greeted him. An emergency room with no receptionist? Someone has to be here. He spun around, surveyed the pandemonium, and zeroed-in on the woman with the clipboard. He rushed toward her, blurting out that he was looking for his son.

Perturbed at being interrupted, she said, "If you haven't found him out here, it means he's already back there." She pointed over her shoulder at the door separating the treatment areas from the waiting room. "Just take a seat and relax."

Smith caught himself searching for an empty seat when he snapped out of this sudden distraction. "My son collapsed on the playground," he said to her. "He was brought here in an ambulance."

"That may be true," the woman acknowledged after a huff. "If it is true, your son is being looked after. Take a seat until your name is called."

"I'm his father!" Smith hissed. "I want to see my son!"

"You'll see the inside of a police car if you continue that kind of verbal abuse."

Pausing to regain his composure, Smith reminded himself that belligerence would get him nowhere. It wasn't right to attack this person, who clearly had too much to do already.

"I'm sorry," he said and returned to the reception window no less determined to find his son but with a better attitude. Arriving there, he met a less official woman wearing sweatpants and a T-shirt as if she'd just come from an aerobics class.

"Universal Coverage Card?" she said, holding out one hand without looking up from the frozen drink she stirred with the other.

Reaching for his wallet, Smith said, "My son was brought here. This is an emergency."

"Like, duh, that's why it's called the emergency room," came the reply.

Insulted by her cavalier response, Smith flushed with anger. He might have said something stern, if not downright ugly, had his finger not touched his Universal Coverage Card.

"Wow," the receptionist remarked as she turned the card over. "This is an original. Haven't seen one in more than five years. Didn't you get a new one in the mail?"

"Listen," Smith said keeping his voice polite but firm, "I'm very worried about my son. Can you make a call or something and see if you can find him?"

After locating her glasses amidst the clutter on her desk, the receptionist told him, "Mr. Smith, you see the crowd out there? Your son has made it through that mess, so I'm sure he's going to be okay."

"I appreciate that but ..."

She held up her hand for him to stop speaking, which infuriated Smith to the point where he was ready to search for Timmy on his own.

"We have, like, a system here." she said. "Give me a few minutes to check around. What's your son's name?"

"Timothy. Timothy Smith," he said deliberately, resisting the temptation to spell it for her.

Rifling through a stack of forms, the receptionist casually sipped her drink and hummed. She might have been flipping through a magazine while she waited her turn at a salon.

Smith's face turned hot as he contemplated his next step. Just then, he caught some movement in the hallway beyond the receptionist's desk. He shifted his gaze, spotted the shape of Hannah's hair, and nearly screamed, "That's my wife!" Instead, he turned away from the window to the door located a few yards to his left. At that moment it opened and someone dressed in scrubs passed into the waiting area.

"Hold that door!" he hollered.

Instantly, the waiting room came to a halt. The running children stopped in their tracks, the crying women fell silent, and every conversation except for the one on the television went dead. The lady with the clipboard stepped sideways to block Smith. She was too late. He slipped by just in time for the door to slam shut on her.

On the other side, Smith found a warren of examination rooms and cubbyhole offices. He followed the hallway where he'd seen Hannah, glancing in any open space he passed. At the end of the hall he turned left again, nearly bowling into his wife who leaned against the wall. Clutching her, he asked what happened to their son.

"They were playing baseball during the afternoon gym class," she replied. Wiping her nose, she continued. "I guess he was running for home plate and just fell down. They thought he tripped or something but then he didn't get up."

Hearing this, Smith suddenly felt his fingers turn cold.

"The kids didn't know what to do. They just told the teacher he fell."

"Tell me he's okay," Smith pleaded.

"I don't know," Hannah blurted and fell against him.

After a few seconds, he asked quietly, "Where is he now?"

"In there with the doctor," Hannah answered. "They told me I couldn't go in."

"You couldn't go in? Why not?"

Smith made for the door to the examination room. His wife smacked his hand away from the knob.

"Parents are only allowed in after the doctor determines there has been no abuse," Hannah explained.

"Abuse? Are you kidding me?"

"Come on, Bob, they have a job to do."

A few seconds later, the door beside Hannah opened. A man wearing a pale blue smock exited the room without so much as a wave to Smith or Hannah. He said, "The nurse explain," as he passed them.

"Wait a minute," Smith called but was distracted by the sight of his son inside the room. It took him a moment to process that Timmy was seated on the table, his legs dangling over the edge. He wasn't laid out under a myriad of equipment nor tended by people dressed for surgery. Only one other person was in the room, presumably a nurse. Smith rushed in and gently embraced his only son.

"Can we go home?" Timmy asked. He wore no shirt, which made it easy for his father to see the reddened skin where tape had once held some type of sensor to the boy's chest.

Smith kept one arm around his son and asked, "How do you feel?"

"I'm fine, dad," Timmy answered. "It was really hot this afternoon; I was sweating like a pig. And I hit a line drive, right past the short stop. Then I stole third and kept going for home."

"Slow down, Timmy," Smith urged. "One play at a time."

"Yeah, so the third baseman dropped the ball and I kept running. I think I was overheated or something and I got real dizzy and just passed out."

"Good. You had us worried," Smith said, making room for Hannah to press her face to their son's cheek.

"You're going to smother the kid," the nurse put in, adding, "When I finish, the boy can wait in the hall while I explain the diagnosis to you." She passed between Hannah and Smith bearing a coarse paper towel. She rubbed Timmy's chest with such vigor that Smith was compelled to pull her hand away.

"Take it easy," he said.

"I know my job," the nurse told him and continued her routine until Timmy's chest was raw. Surveying her work, she said, "Now you can step outside so I can talk to your designated guardians."

At the sound of this term, Timmy screwed up his face. He said, "They're my mom and dad."

"Says you. Let's go," the nurse told him.

"Where's his shirt?" Smith asked.

It was the nurse's turn to produce a funny face. "I'm not in charge of laundry," she replied.

Smith removed his own oxford and helped Timmy slip his arms into it. After buttoning the shirt, he told his son to wait just outside the door, that he would be out in a minute.

When Timmy was outside the nurse closed the door with a firm hand and faced his parents. "The doctor has determined that your son probably has a defective heart valve," she informed them. "The cause of his collapse was most likely the backflow of un-oxygenated blood."

Smith and Hannah expected some sort of unremarkable malady along the lines of a kid who simply exhausted himself. This news left them breathless. Such a diagnosis sounded like something for an old man who smoked his whole life not one for a boy who was a star athlete and who just left the room under his own power.

"You're sure?" Smith croaked.

"The doctor made this determination," the nurse replied.

As an engineer, Smith believed in empirical evidence, in proven results. It was this type of thinking that took over when he asked, "What tests did he run?"

"Are you a doctor, Mr. Smith?" the nurse questioned.

"I'm an engineer," Smith retorted, "not that it matters. I'd like to know what tests were performed. I'd like to talk to the doctor."

"I would like an extra day off each month," the nurse put in. "We don't always get what we want."

Before Smith could challenge that comment, the lecture continued.

"Timothy Smith should avoid any strenuous activity. His school nurse will be notified by a Care Delivery Specialist, who should be here doing what I'm doing, but the facility is understaffed today. Anyway, the designated CDS will explain the case to Timothy's school nurse, as well as any academic or physical requirements from which he will be exempt as provided under the Universal Healthcare and Medical Assistance Act. The nurse will be required to develop a contingency plan should Timothy's condition present itself during school hours."

"Hold on a second," Smith said. "What are we supposed to do right now? I mean, is Timmy well enough to go home? Should he stay here?"

"Mr. Smith, your son might live a completely normal life."

"Might?"

"That's right, he could outgrow the problem. The doctor said that he should be monitored for ninety days, after which you should schedule a visit to your Primary Care Clinic for further evaluation."

Nodding, Smith said, "But he collapsed on the playground. He was unconscious, wasn't he?"

"That's why he's not to engage in strenuous activity. It increases the likelihood that his heart will malfunction."

"You talk about him like he's an old car or something."

"For the sake of clarity, Mr. Smith, we use technical terms. Upon discharge of the client, you'll be given a package of care recommendations. I strongly suggest you follow them to the letter."

"We will," Smith said, "but shouldn't he stay here for observation or more tests?"

The nurse folded her arms. "Let's put this in perspective. Timothy's condition is no longer an emergency. The doctor gave your son a thorough examination, determined the most likely cause of his collapse, and has prescribed a reasonable course of action. Timothy walked out of this room on his own two feet with no assistance."

"She's right," Hannah chimed in.

He took a couple seconds to compose himself before saying, "This *is* a serious condition, isn't it?"

"It can be. Set an appointment with your Primary Care Clinic so that Timothy will be in the system. It's the best thing to do."

"Thank you," Hannah said. "Would it be possible to talk to the doctor anyway, or maybe get a second opinion? We're just worried about our son."

In a lower tone the nurse answered, "The Universal Coverage Contract entitles you to a second opinion with administrative approval."

CHAPTER TWO

THE LOOK ON HIS DAD'S FACE frightened Timmy more than waking up in the emergency room with that strange man staring at him. He saw that his dad was angry but also confused, an expression that rarely clouded his features. And his mother appeared to be plain dumbstruck, like his classmate, Jill, when the teacher asked her to name the capital of Minnesota.

Timmy remembered hitting that line drive, really connecting with the ball the way Coach Dolante taught him. He could recall the groan of the third baseman when the ball bounced out of his glove. The next thing he knew he was flat on his back with a stranger peering at him. He felt cold and tired, as if he'd been swimming on a breezy day and didn't have a towel. The stranger probed his body, stuck several spongy discs to his chest, and uttered strange words with a sing-song lilt to another person who was out of sight. It was like being in a scary movie.

Sometime later, the discs were yanked off and he was escorted to the room where his parents showed up a few minutes later. The nurse came in after a nasty exchange with his mom. Though he couldn't see her, he knew it was his mother by the sound of her voice, and Timmy nearly ran out after her. He couldn't do that without looking like a sissy and he was a champion, or at least a champion in the making. His coach said so.

What upset him most was that the nurse's eye sockets were misaligned to the point where he couldn't be sure if she was tilting her head or if he was losing his balance. He resorted to staring at the floor, which didn't suit her. She cupped his chin with a fat hand, admonishing him not to be scared.

He nearly slapped her hand away when she touched him the second time. He wasn't scared and the only reason he didn't knock her hand off was because his father had taught him to respect professional people who were all supposed to be smart and helpful. The trouble was, this lady seemed to be neither. However, Timmy did as he was told, hoping that his dad would arrive soon to get him out of there.

Then the doctor came in and listened to Timmy's heart through a stethoscope before tucking the instrument into his pocket with a shrug. The nurse handed him a form which he scribbled on in handwriting that the boy knew would never have passed his father's critical eye. His dad insisted he shape every letter perfectly on his homework. "Words are like buildings," Timmy heard him say a hundred times. "They have to stand up straight." Teachers thought he was showing off, but he was actually pleasing his dad when he wrote out his spelling list in a precise hand.

Finally, his dad came out of the room, appearing somewhat satisfied but still a bit angry or confused. It was difficult for Timmy to discern which one it was. He was bewildered himself since no one told him what happened on the playground, if he'd fallen and hit his head or if he'd crashed into another kid and knocked himself out. He told his dad it was the heat but maybe it was something else.

Timmy didn't like his parents having a private conversation with the nurse. It wasn't fair. It made him feel stupid, and judging by the straight A's he earned on every report card, he wasn't stupid. What's more, his dad's shirt hung off him like a Halloween costume. If one of his pals saw him like this he'd never hear the end of it.

Still, when his father's arm fell over his shoulders, Timmy straightened up and got into step. He wouldn't let his dad down. He would show him that the nurse wasn't scary, nor was the doctor or this whole experience. Whatever they had talked about, his dad would tell him the truth. He'd be back on the field tomorrow, hitting home runs, stealing bases, and leading his team to victory.

"We're going home, son," his dad said. "You'll be just fine."

Despite this admonition, the Smith family couldn't leave immediately. First, they had to complete the paperwork and the receptionist was no longer in a good humor. Her frozen drink stood to the side, a melted mess of coagulated chocolate, and she was not humming a pleasant tune either. She handed Smith a Treatment Rendered Receipt, stabbing it with her chubby finger. As Smith put his signature on the line, he offered an apologetic smile but the receptionist ignored it. She next handed him a sheaf of papers that included the doctor's preliminary recommended care scheme, something called Primary Cardiac Care and Advisories. Smith initialed a receipt for it as well.

"Be sure to get a current Universal Coverage Card, Mr. Smith. Your card may not be accepted the next time you require service."

"I'll do that," he said contritely. He saw a red placard screwed into the wall just beneath the window that separated her from the boisterous waiting room.

MEDICAL EMERGENCY FUEL VOUCHERS MUST BE STAMPED.

He waited a moment to be sure there were no more papers coming from the other side of the desk. Then, he cleared his throat gently and asked if the receptionist might provide him with just such a voucher.

Like an old boiler, she puffed and wheezed before finally extracting the form from the bottom drawer in her desk. She stared at it, weighing whether or not Smith deserved one. His earlier impatience had been an affront to her sensibilities and was cause for a categorical denial. After a final look over her glasses at the cute boy who had the misfortune to be this man's son, she curled her fingers around the red stamp. The kid was going to be swarmed with girls in a couple years, just as soon as he showed those first hints of manhood. She smacked the stamp onto the voucher like a sledgehammer. Nonetheless, the pale ink was barely visible. She handed it to Smith and reached for the next set of paperwork without looking at him again.

"Thank you," Smith said and turned for the door, his wife and son in his wake.

Low on fuel, Smith told Hannah to head home with Timmy, that he would be there soon. Before they split up he hugged his son one more time.

Arriving at Delaware County Fuel Depot Number 3, Smith parked his pickup in an open spot. The stamped voucher folded neatly in his pocket, he stood in line behind ten other people, all of them following a procedure which required that their voucher first be verified by a clerk before they were given a matching electronic chit that was subsequently surrendered to the Transfer Technician who actually dispensed fuel into their vehicle. All of this was overseen by a pair of pistol-bearing Federal Energy Security Bureau policemen. No one moved their car from the holding pen to the pumps without a nod from the attending cops. In the early days of the system there had been fights as people jockeyed to get their allotment of gas. Hence the policemen, who had the power to deny anyone access for the smallest infraction.

Smith was surprised to see a line this early in the afternoon. He surveyed those ahead of him. Each wore the harried but bored look of people frustrated at having to wait for no good reason. Smith caught his own reflection in the window, noting that his expression, while somewhat relieved, still showed the stress of his visit to the emergency room. He released a nervous cough, told himself that Timmy was going to be fine, and moved one step closer to the door.

When Smith finally went inside to get his chit, he was passed by an older man using a sturdy wooden cane. He wore an open shirt with rolled-up sleeves. The man caught Smith's eye and gave him a wink.

"These dolts test my patience most every time," the man said in a bold voice, his chit pinched between his fingertips.

No one spoke this way at a fueling depot, especially not within earshot of the clerks who verified vouchers and authorized chits. Smith resisted the urge to react, averting his eyes in case one of the employees thought he agreed with the sentiment. While he thought the process should operate a bit faster, he understood the necessity of it. Without controlling systems there was simply too much room for fraud and profiteering.

The man continued outside under the gaze of those still in line. They watched him walk across the holding pen where he exchanged words with one of the policemen. The cop pointed a stiff finger in an unpleasant way at a pickup parked in the pen.

Everyone returned their attention to the clerk, who glared with contempt that they had not moved forward on their own.

Smith's turn finally came. He presented his voucher through the slot beneath the bulletproof window separating him from the clerk on the other side. It took several minutes for the barcode on the voucher to be scanned into the computer, a chit to be coded, the clerk to sign and stamp the voucher with the Fuel Depot's official mark, and add his initials within the stamp's border. Then Smith's receipt and chit were stuffed through the slot.

Like a yawning hippo, the clerk tilted his head back and hollered, "NEXT!"

Outside, Smith walked to his vehicle less annoyed by the clerk's imperious behavior than he was grateful to have another seven gallons of gas. It was more than he burned going to and from the hospital. Now he might have a little extra to take Timmy somewhere.

As he arrived at the side of his pickup he saw that the man who mouthed off about the clerk was leaning against his own truck just a few spaces away. Smith couldn't help but admire the way it gleamed under what had to be a fresh coat of wax. With several cars ahead of him and having always been fond of pickups, he ambled over for a closer look.

"Beautiful," Smith said.

"Chevrolet Silverado, this one being the last of the breed," came the man's reply. "Your father used to do all the maintenance for me."

"My father?" Smith queried. Then it struck him. The man was Doctor Ben, a regular at his father's old service station.

"Wow, I haven't seen you in ..."

Doctor Ben finished the sentence with, "... perhaps twenty years."

"Almost," Smith reflected, impressed with Ben's memory. He put out his hand and said, "Sorry I didn't recognize you in there."

"Not a problem. You were headed off to Drexel. Engineering, wasn't it?"

"I'm the foundation team leader," Smith replied, "at Wexler Associates."

"Excellent. Wife? Kids?"

"One of each. Hannah and Timmy."

"I take that to mean you're all together."

"We are," Smith answered with pride. After a breath he added, "I'm on my way home from the hospital. My son was taken to the emergency room."

Ben's face showed immediate concern. "Forgive me, my bedside manner is a little rusty. How's your boy doing?"

"Well enough, I suppose. The doctor says he has a defective heart valve."

"Hmmmm," Doctor Ben murmured. "Where do you live?"

"In Cliffwood, just above Media."

"So they took your son to Media General?"

"That's right."

"You're out of my district," Doctor Ben said, "but if I'm in the area, I'll stop by and take a look at your son." He fished into his pocket and produced a business card.

Smith took the card, reading, Visiting Physician, District 128. "I would appreciate that," he said. "Nothing against the doctor in the emergency room, but I'm going to get a second opinion."

"Always a good idea. We doctors are human, and we make mistakes."

Smith couldn't help but hope that the emergency room doctor had made an error in his diagnosis. The last thing he wanted for his son was a serious operation, one that might endanger his life even if it was part of the cure.

"Let's go!" called the policeman standing at the pen's gate.

"Hark! The herald angels sing," Ben mocked him. "Take care of yourself and your son, Bob. If you need anything, give me a call. Don't let arbitrary lines drawn on a map scare you off."

"Thank you," Smith said and walked back to his truck. He watched Ben roll past the cop without so much as a tap on the brakes. Is that the type of guy he'd want to examine his son? He wasn't sure and yet there was a certain appeal to him. His eyes showed as much confidence as his voice, and while he used the cane to assist his right leg, he moved with all the purpose and menace of a grizzly bear. In normal circumstances these qualities might not have been enticing, but in an emergency, as Smith had just faced, it would be nice to have someone who asserted himself.

Waiting his turn, Smith ruminated over what the nurse had told him. He wanted to believe that a mistake had been made, that the test results were erroneous or that the doctor misinterpreted them. He'd seen this in his own profession, an honest mistake of man or machine that could be corrected or revised.

Of course, what frustrated Smith most was his dependency.

He couldn't order new tests or consult another doctor in a hurry and thereby have a definitive result. He was a senior engineer with the authority to make such things happen at Wexler Associates. However, there was a system in place for medical care. It was called Universal Coverage. It guaranteed care to every citizen, as well as to those individuals who found themselves inside the borders. This system had its own administrators, who like Smith in his field, made the decisions as to what tests were performed or not.

Hearing a whistle, Smith raised his eyes to see the cop waving at him. He got behind the wheel and drove toward the pumps.

"I'm kinda tired, dad," Timmy said, greeting his father at the door.

"It's been a tough day," Smith replied. "Why don't you take a nap? I'll wake you in an hour or so for supper."

Satisfied that Timmy was out of earshot, Smith sat with Hannah across the corner of the kitchen table. His mind was suddenly overwhelmed by everything that had happened. One minute he was meeting the President of the United States and the next he was speeding to the hospital. First he was told his son might die; then he was informed he might outgrow the affliction. A vision of his son dead at the age of eleven competed with one of him hitting the winning home run for the World Champion Philadelphia Phillies. Of all the things he figured might happen in the course of Timmy's childhood, he never imagined that a defective heart valve would crop up.

"We have to get a second opinion," he said to Hannah.

Hannah blew out a lungful of air. "Maybe we should do what the nurse told us," she suggested.

"We're going to, and we're also going to get him to another doctor. Quick. This is his heart we're talking about, not a skinned knee."

"He might outgrow it," Hannah said hopefully. "The nurse said so."

"I don't want to think about what will happen if he doesn't. Besides, we have Universal Coverage in this country. Let's find a specialist and get him fixed up right."

"Have you seen that book lately?"

"No," Smith admitted. In fact, he'd hardly opened the Universal Coverage Manual. Every year it came to the house, landing on the doorstep the way the Yellow Pages used to. In the age of virtual information, he couldn't understand why trees were killed to print this book. Then again, he knew the answer. Not everyone had a computer or access to one. Thus, the UCM, as it was known, would be available for immediate consultation, which was only fair to the less fortunate who probably needed it most.

"Where is it?" he asked.

Hannah did him the favor of retrieving it from the bottom of the hall closet. She flopped the monstrous book onto the table with a thud then went to the sink for a cloth to wipe off the dust. Smith waited patiently. He was in no hurry to scour through this reference volume. Like every one of its kind, he figured there were only a few useful pieces of information that pertained to his situation. The trick was finding them without wasting the entire day.

It took him an hour and a half.

He started logically, with the table of contents, read through the Client Bill of Rights, and continued on to the Standards of Care to Be Provided. He finished with Procedures for Second Opinions. As he closed the UCM cover, he realized he was alone at the table. Hannah abandoned him for the living room couch, which faced the television. She never missed the evening news.

Smith approached his wife with his analysis. "We're getting a second opinion," he began.

"Is that you sitting behind the President?" Hannah asked with her finger pointed at the TV.

Smith squinted at the screen. The camera showed the President making his speech earlier that day. To the left sat Smith, Mark Wexler, and the rest of the people who had been in the conference room.

"That's me," he said jovially. "I met him later, too."

"You met the President of the United States!" Hannah exclaimed.

"Shhh. Timmy's resting," he admonished her. "It was just a handshake, that's all."

"Still," Hannah whispered, "You got to meet him. I remember when he ran the first time."

Smith did, too. He and Hannah first encountered each other at a rally on the University of Pennsylvania's campus, where she had been a student and he a visitor from Drexel.

From the television there came a cheer, but Hannah muted the volume and inquired about Timmy's second opinion.

"We have to get administrative approval for the second opinion, which should be no problem. The UCM says that in cases of certain diagnoses, a second opinion is automatically considered. One of us has to go to the Health Administration District Office with the paperwork they gave us at the hospital. With an approved second opinion, Timmy can see a specialist. That person will lay out our options."

"What does that mean?"

"I'm not a doctor," Smith said, "but I know valve replacement surgery is nothing new."

"Valve replacement surgery?" Hannah repeated, horrified by the idea that her son's chest would be cut open.

"I don't know, honey. We'll have to see what the specialist says."

They both pondered the calamity they now faced.

Hannah had the final word. "I can't imagine what this is going to cost," she said. "We're lucky to have Universal Coverage."

They agreed it was best if he took Timmy for a walk, an easy one, after supper. The two of them would have a father and son chat about the situation. A sample script for this conversation was in the UCM under the section: HOW TO TELL SIGNIFICANT OTHERS ABOUT THE WORST. Smith didn't see it as quite that bad, but he read the dialog, filling in the appropriate blanks as he did. He felt confident that he could do the job, which required him to tell the truth without alarming Timmy.

As the UCM recommended, the family ate a favorite meal of the afflicted person's choosing. Timmy loved meatloaf, and Hannah baked one using low-fat turkey instead of hamburger. Halfway through the meal, no one seemed to remember that they had all been to the emergency room earlier in the day. Smith kept his story about the President to himself. It would only diminish the importance of the matter at hand, which according to the UCM was that the afflicted person have some enjoyment.

Timmy rattled on about his classmates, whom he had bested in a spelling contest. Smith congratulated his son and reminded him to keep his letters straight and even. Then Timmy drew his name in the sauce stain on his plate using a knife. Smith underlined it then poked his fork into the remaining piece of meatloaf. His son squealed and Smith gave it back with a laugh. While cheerful through these antics, Hannah appeared slightly distant, like a stage director observing her actors. She offered to clear the table, thereby giving Smith the opportunity to leave with Timmy.

Outside, father and son headed down the sidewalk. Cliffwood was the name of the development, which made no sense given that the land was a rolling plain with no sign of any cliffs. It was just a catchy name the developer invented to comfort people about the prices they paid for the houses. It was also congruous with a similar collection of nearby homes bearing the name Briarwood.

As he moved along, Smith's consternation expanded to another subject. He noted that several houses on his street remained empty. His former neighbors moved out more than two years ago. Living in the suburbs wasn't what it used to be. Expensive transportation was the problem. Gasoline cost more than ten dollars a gallon, if you had an approved voucher to buy it. Everyone carpooled or used mass transit to get to work. Leisure trips to the mall or the movies or a restaurant required serious planning.

As he walked with Timmy at his side, he couldn't help but remember how he came to live in this neighborhood. He and Hannah worked in the city, but she was insistent on getting out of their "two-box" apartment, a reference to the one bedroom, one bathroom place they'd rented after getting married while he was a grad student.

"What have we been saving for?" she asked one night.

"But we're so close to school," Smith replied.

"And everyone else. This place reeks like the Korean restaurant on the corner."

On some days, the kitchen exhaust fan did send odd scents into their open windows. There was noise, too, especially from a couple four doors down who liked to bring their arguments into the hallway.

"One of these days I'm going to step off the elevator and get hit with a flying lamp or something," Hannah said. "Then what?"

During a particularly busy month, Smith told her to find them a house of their own. He hadn't been serious; he'd only wanted to get her off his back so he could concentrate. She took a week's vacation, rented a car, and roamed three counties in search of a dream home. She found the perfect one. Whether he'd been serious or not, he was about to move.

"It's in a gated community," she'd said, "but it doesn't look like an ant farm. Every house is different."

Every house was different, designed by a team of architects who knew how to reverse, flip, and rotate a common floor plan. To add cachet, they varied the styles of kitchen cabinets, crown moldings, and floor coverings. Smith, with his engineer's eye, knew the tricks of the trade and was not deceived. Still, he surrendered to his wife's desire and emptied the savings account his father had started for him when he was Timmy's age.

"Save this for a place of your own," his father had said every time they went to the bank to make a deposit.

Smith had added steadily to that account. Money flowed in from after-school and summer jobs, birthday cards, and soon to be deceased aunts. Then there was the substantial signing bonus from Wexler Associates, enough to give him visions of owning a penthouse. In addition, he automatically transferred ten percent of his salary to savings. By the time they moved in and bought a few pieces of furniture, the account had to be closed for lack of funds. The direct savings deposits were channeled to higher utility bills.

"We need vehicles," Hannah had said one night over the new

kitchen table. The dining room contained nothing atop its perfectly vacuumed carpet. "Can't your dad find us a good deal?"

Eventually, his father found him a used pickup, which Smith knew would be handy for the inevitable projects that would come up around the house. Hannah disagreed.

"That's the best your father could find?" she asked upon seeing it parked in the driveway.

"It's a work in progress," Smith told her.

The next day she bought a brand new coupe for herself on a no-money-down basis and her good credit.

The first few years in the new house couldn't have been better, especially when Timmy came along. Smith's father restored the pickup to nearly new status. Hannah worked as an administrator at the University of Pennsylvania, while Smith climbed a few rungs of the ladder at Wexler.

It was this point in his life that Smith thought had been the best. Hannah took a leave of absence to nurse Timmy. Smith strengthened his reputation with Mr. Wexler by executing challenging projects in record time. He logged more hours than anyone on his floor and was paid accordingly. The house filled with furniture, Hannah traded her car for a sport utility vehicle with the safest crash test ratings, and the three of them took a well-deserved vacation to Florida.

Then his father fell ill. He deteriorated steadily despite various treatments and surgeries.

"These new doctors," his father said, "they're wasting my time just so they can collect a buck."

This wasn't true, and Smith reminded his father that they were trying to save his life.

"Save my life?" protested his father. "We're all gonna die, Bob."

Smith had meant they were trying to prolong his life, to make it more comfortable, and his father knew it.

"Bullshit," came the response. "They're on this new program with the government. This Universal Coverage thing or whatever it's called. They get paid as long as they keep me kicking. When I'm done, they have to stop billing Uncle Sam."

This reference to the recently instituted Universal Coverage System was not lost on Smith. He didn't like his father's criticism, especially because the man was benefiting directly from it. He and Hannah had worked tirelessly for the presidential candidate whose platform included healthcare for everyone. The same man was still president since the repeal of the 22nd Amendment allowed him to run for a third term, and millions of people like Smith and Hannah voted for him.

"You're getting a good deal," Smith had said to his father, proud of what he and Hannah had done during that election year. They went door to door to all the apartment buildings in their area, handing out pamphlets to everyone except the fighting couple down the hall. They spent hours registering students on both campuses. In the end, it made a difference. Their man won by a landslide; he had a mandate, which included Universal Coverage among many other things.

Smith's father had smiled at his son's optimism. "That's for damn sure. The taxes I paid for this don't amount to a quarter inch wrench on a two-inch bolt. You'll be stuck with the balance, son. I can guarantee that. When your turn comes there's not going to a be a dime left in the piggybank."

"Knock if off, dad," was all Smith could say.

"Find that army doc," his father said. "The one who patched me up in the Gulf War. Yanked out a couple pieces of shrapnel, scraped me clean, dumped some antiseptic in the holes, and I was good as new. If he says I'm done, then I'll go home and save the taxpayers some money. How's that sound?"

"I think you should listen to what the doctors here tell you and stop being a pain in the ass."

"Bah! Your mother never called me that, God rest her soul. I wish I had gone first."

"Please, dad."

From that day things slowly changed in ways Smith neither expected nor understood. Hannah went back to work, leaving Timmy in the care of a nanny. The first one was a thief, the second one incompetent, the third one a slob. A fourth woman, Nadzia, from Poland of all places, was fantastic but she completed her nursing studies and moved on. They didn't seek a fifth because by then Timmy was in school most of the day.

The local schools were another of Hannah's reasons for demanding the particular house they purchased. The district in which it was located was famous for its advanced programs, not to mention the sports teams. Their son would have every opportunity to grow up a well-rounded person. They couldn't deny him that and claim to be decent parents.

The changes continued and they were no longer confined to Smith's small piece of the world. There was a global financial crisis that dissipated into a recession, which lingered for a few years before the economy melted down completely. The public came to understand what the word depression meant in economic terms. Initially, the price of oil plummeted but soon hit record highs when another war in the Middle East began with Iran's closure of the Straits of Hormuz. By the time it ended four years later, the shattered world economy looked as if it would never recover.

Fuel of every type was rationed in the United States for the first time since World War II. Congressional committees declared the country was not to be held hostage by greedy oil barons. The government nationalized the oil industry to prevent profiteering. While private companies nominally operated the production and distribution of petroleum products, they were under the aegis of the Federal Energy Regulatory Commission. The Federal Government itself retained a fifty-one percent stake in every major corporation involved in the business, having given back the other forty-nine percent to the original shareholders.

One of those shareholders had been Smith's father, the owner of a typical corner gas station. Through an incentive program, he had accumulated shares in the company that supplied him with the gasoline he sold. The station had a loyal following, especially among working women who liked to have the old-fashioned service of an attendant who pumped the gas and checked their oil. The price was the same so there was no reason to go anywhere else. The elder Smith stuck to the repair bays while young men in crisp blue shirts operated the pumps. Those young men dispensed record amounts of fuel for the size of the station. Their boss was rewarded with a monthly share bonus.

"That's Exxon-Mobil," Smith's father said. "You can take it to the bank." He requested the certificates themselves, eventually collecting a stack of them that filled a heavy manila envelope.

Robert Smith, the bereaved son who inherited those certificates, found that he owned less than one share for every two his father had earned thanks to the government takeover during the war. He also paid a heavy estate tax on that legacy, which left him with about a quarter of his father's intended gift. He kept a single certificate as a memento. It hung at home on the wall beside his desk.

As he paused to cross the street with Timmy, he remembered what happened to the money that came from the other shares. He used it to pay off Hannah's SUV, which seemed like a good idea at the time. Now he wished he had the money for Timmy's future.

Smith forced himself to think about the happier times. There was the joy of being a father, of watching his son grow up. Timmy was an enthusiastic student, energetic, and not prone to trouble. He led his pals more than he followed them, something that impressed Smith when he watched them play their games on the Little League field. Smith came to appreciate his own father's efforts in raising him. His father welcomed him into his neighborhood garage even as he encouraged the young Smith to get a college education. In this way, he had the best of both worlds: hands-on experience and theoretical training. He looked forward to sharing the same knowledge with Timmy.

The trouble was this bad heart valve, and the time had come to tell Timmy about it.

"I spoke with the nurse in the hospital today," Smith began.

"She was weird looking, dad."

"That's not nice, Timmy. She's a professional, a person who spent years learning her skills. Don't judge a person by their looks. Judge them by their talent. Coach Dolante picked you because you out-slugged those other boys didn't he?"

"Yeah, but she was kind of mean. She almost scraped my skin off."

This was true but Smith decided to let it go. "The thing is, Timmy, there's a reason you fell down on the playground today."

Timmy kicked his foot at the sidewalk. "I know. I was running so hard."

"There's more to it than that. The doctor did some tests on you and he discovered something."

Instinctively, Timmy touched one of the sore spots on his

chest. He could not remember if there had been wires or not. Whatever the case, having had a nap and supper, he felt as well as any day in his life. He was ready to step up to the plate and hit a homer.

"Remember when I explained how a car engine works?" Smith asked his son.

"Yeah."

"The valves open and close at different times ..."

"I remember," Timmy interrupted.

"Well, your heart also has valves that open and close."

"They taught us that in health class."

Smith was pleased to hear this. "Just like a car engine, the valves have to open and close tightly and at the right times."

Without realizing it, Timmy slowed his pace. At first he couldn't imagine anything was wrong, but his father was giving him a serious and detailed explanation. He knew that whenever his father used this tone it was about something important, something he should know and remember.

"One of the valves in your heart is a little sticky," Smith finally said. He nearly choked at the sound of his own words.

"Sticky?" Timmy asked.

"According to the doctor, you have a valve that stays open a little when it should be closed."

"Nah," the younger Smith said. His father spoke carefully, which meant this might be a test of some kind, like those pop quizzes Mrs. Marselek liked to give on Thursdays.

Nodding at his son's rebuttal, Smith held back for several paces. He caught himself forming a detailed explanation of the human circulatory system. It was the engineer in him again. Now was not the time to be an engineer but rather a father.

"Your mother and I are going to take you to some more doctors, Timmy. These doctors are going to check you out. They're going to see if your heart valve needs to get tuned up or if it's fine just the way it is. Do you understand?"

"Dad, I'm the fastest kid on the field. I'm playing Little League this summer."

Smith put his arm around Timmy and pulled him into his hip. "You're going to be a champion, son."

"I am, dad. I know I am."

CHAPTER THREE

SMITH AND TIMMY ARRIVED HOME to find Hannah on the couch. She exchanged a look with her husband, who replied with a subtle rocking of his head. Neither discussed the topic of Timmy's care until their son had gone to bed. Even then, they waited half an hour not because they thought he might be a while getting to sleep but because they didn't know where to start.

At last Smith took his turn. He said, "Someone has to take this paperwork to school with Timmy so the principal knows what's going on."

"I can do that," Hannah offered. "I'll give Dean Simon a call and tell him I'll be in late." Simon was director of admissions at the University of Pennsylvania, Hannah's alma mater. She'd been working with him since completing her degree there.

"One of us has to go to the Health Administration District Office," Smith continued, "to get a second opinion authorized."

"I don't even know where it is."

"The address is in the UC Manual."

"Can't we call?"

"Apparently not. They require a personal visit, probably to prevent fraud or something."

"Are we supposed to take a day off work to do this? I mean, Dean Simon has begun assigning interviews. I have ten a day this week and we're just getting started."

Smith appreciated her workload. He faced a similar dilemma at Central West. It was the most important job in the Wexler portfolio. Although his team functioned well on their own, he didn't want a mistake to slip through, not with all the politicians watching so closely. The first part of the project was the foundation and if anything went wrong it might put the whole development in jeopardy. At a minimum, Wexler Associates and Smith's team would look stupid.

Seeing the dread on her husband's face, Hannah slid close to him on the couch. "Look," she said, placing a gentle kiss on his lips then pulling away. "We're panicking. We need to step back, gain some perspective, and not let our fears get the best of us."

These words came to Smith in the soothing voice he remembered from their early dates. Hannah had been a sociology major and now applied those skills to selecting Penn's future students. Sure, she had a dramatic streak in her that came out from time to time, but she had evolved into an even-keeled sort of woman who reserved her passion for things that truly mattered. He appreciated her ability to adapt, as he was prone to worry about too many details, a quality that made him a good engineer.

"After I talk to Timmy's homeroom teacher and the principal," Hannah continued, "I'll check with the nurse to make sure the Care Delivery Specialist gave her instructions about our son. Then I'll call you with an update that will put you at ease."

"That should do it," Smith acknowledged.

"Exactly. In the meantime, you can put in a request to human resources for a day off to get the second opinion approval. The UCM guarantees Certified Caregivers paid leave."

"Certified Caregivers?"

Using her toe, Hannah nudged the UCM on the coffee table. "It's in there," she said. "The best part is the Certified Caregiver application is online. I'll have it done for both of us before Monday morning."

She must have read about this while I was out with Timmy, Smith thought. Furthermore, it was good news. He couldn't remember if that provision had been incorporated into Universal Coverage or not. Hannah was telling him that it was and he would benefit from it. He took comfort knowing that his paycheck would be the same, regardless of whether he or Hannah missed a day here and there to take Timmy to the doctor. He recalled a television commercial from the election. In it, a single mother lamented the fact that her boss had cut her pay because she took her little girl to the hospital. The woman was living paycheck to paycheck. Because of the pay cut, she couldn't make her rent and ended up in a homeless shelter. Smith wasn't close to that situation, but neither did he have a flush savings account. In fact, he only had the money in his checkbook, which was enough to cover the family's expenses for a couple of months. He'd been meaning to save more and starting this week he would.

"We can't delay this," he said.

"We're not delaying it," Hannah insisted. "We're doing what

we can as fast as we can. Don't forget what the nurse told us: Timmy needs to take it easy. I'll make that clear at school, and we'll both keep an eye on him here at home."

"You better believe it," Smith confirmed.

"We've got the best doctors in the world right here in Philadelphia. One of them will take a look at Timmy, and in no time he'll be right as rain."

"We do have good doctors here, don't we?"

"The best care possible," Hannah finished, repeating the Universal Coverage motto as she scooped up the remote and switched the channel to her favorite program.

The tension of the day drained out of Smith. He stared at the television without comprehending the program. Images and sounds floated past him as daydreams of his own childhood blended with memories of times spent with Timmy. An hour or so later, he surrendered the couch for his bed.

On the way down the hall he peeked into Timmy's room. To Smith's surprise, his son's eyes were open, staring at him from across the room.

"Am I going to be okay, dad?" he asked.

"You have nothing to worry about," Smith said. "Take it easy the way I told you, alright?"

"I want to be a champion."

"You already are. Do your homework and study and you'll be a smart one, too."

•◆• •◆• •◆•

The weekend passed with Smith struggling to keep Timmy off the baseball field.

"I'm gonna suck if I don't practice," Timmy complained.

"A champion doesn't use that kind of language, son."

"Nothing hurts! I should be on the field."

"Why don't you catch up on your reading," Smith suggested.

"School's over in a couple weeks."

"School's not over for three weeks, and before you know it, the summer semester will start."

"Joey's dad said when he was a kid he didn't have school in the summer. Why do we have to go?"

"Because it's good for you," Smith replied. An overwhelming majority of voters supported the Summer Education Enhancement Referendum. It was beneficial for everyone: kids with learning disabilities had extra time to finish the year's work; other kids enjoyed electives like music and foreign languages; and parents avoided the cost of daycare. Teachers' unions supported the initiative after Congress appropriated federal money to pay a proportionate salary for months they normally weren't in the classroom.

Monday morning arrived with Josh in Smith's driveway exactly on time. Over the past decade, they worked together on various projects at Wexler and shared transportation responsibilities once energy rationing was imposed. Josh lived only half a mile away in Briarwood. He and Smith alternately drove to the local Far Area Rapid Transit Station in Media or to the office. This saved them hundreds of dollars and gave them a tax credit in the bargain.

"How did things turn out with Timmy?" Josh asked.

"We'll see," Smith replied.

"That bad."

"Like everything, a second opinion is required."

"It'll work out. Kids are tough; they bounce back."

"You're right," Smith said, wondering if he really believed

that. Switching on the radio, he nearly chuckled at the memory of listening to traffic reports. How many times had he tuned the pickup's radio to the news station for just that purpose? Looking ahead at the sparsely traveled road he realized that driving to work had never been easier. Of course it had never been as expensive. Ten dollar a gallon gasoline, six hundred dollar annual vehicle registration fees, and an exorbitant parking tax all made driving a luxury. He could afford it thanks to his position as foundation team leader at Wexler Associates. Yet, on Mondays, they only drove about three miles to the FART station in Media. To both of them, the environment was more important than the money.

As Smith noted the night before, people were leaving the suburbs for the city. He would have preferred to stay there after earning his graduate degree, but Hannah insisted on a house. Truth be told, after seeing the one she picked, he'd wanted out of the city, too. Yes, the house was a cookie cutter variation of those around it, but it shared walls, odors, and arguments with no one. There was a garage and a backyard and a quiet street in front where Smith imagined his children learning to ride their bikes. He happily signed the mortgage.

Cruising along in the passenger seat, he told himself this had not been a mistake. Who could have predicted another war? Rationing? Are you kidding? Things like that didn't happen in the United States.

And then they did.

Without realizing it, Smith had arrived at the train station. He'd been distracted between his worries about Timmy and memories of the past. The front tires bumped the stop in their parking space but Smith made no move to get out of the car.

"You staying here?" Josh asked with a grin.

"Sorry," Smith replied and released his seat belt.

"Let's hope the train gets us there before lunch."

In uncharacteristic fashion, the FART ran without a single delay. After a few minutes' ride on the subway, Smith and Josh walked the last four blocks to the Wexler building.

Smith's legs ached as he climbed ten flights of stairs to the floor he shared with dozens of his co-workers. Josh bounded ahead of him, asking if Smith wanted him to wait.

"Go ahead," Smith said, pausing on the landing for the Seventh Floor. He refused to sit down, but he clutched the railing and struggled to catch his breath. Panic as much as fatigue suddenly caught hold of him. He contemplated the consequences of Timmy collapsing on the playground a second time. What if it happened today, a day when he didn't have a vehicle? What if the ambulance didn't get there in time? His son might die alone among strangers. Smith squeezed the railing until his fingers faded to white.

"Do you want to stop off on eight for a coffee?"

Smith turned from the wall to see Ralph, another co-worker, coming up the stairs.

"Come on, boss. You know when the elevators are off we get another ten minutes to log in," Ralph said. "Besides, the coffee's free."

Sweating as he was from the effort of climbing the stairs and the stress of Timmy's condition, hot coffee was the last thing Smith wanted to drink. "I'll pass," he replied.

"Your loss," Ralph commented on his way up the next flight. "Just remember, Wexler's getting rich keeping those elevators off longer than he has to."

These last words floated down the stairwell to Smith who

spun his head as Ralph's shoes went around the corner of the landing above.

"Hang on a second," Smith called as he found the energy to go after Ralph. "What's this about the elevators being off longer than they have to be?"

Ralph reached for the door accessing the eighth floor and smirked over his shoulder. "Think about it. Wexler gets credit for the net energy not used. You and I and every other schlub in this building puffs up the stairs while Wexler rakes in the cash."

"That doesn't make any sense," Smith countered. "The company is only allowed so many kilowatts."

"Yeah, and when we make sure the company uses less by humping up and down these stairs, he gets a tax credit. Do the math, Bob. A tax credit equals more money in Wexler's pocket, not ours. He's using us to make more money and we're not getting paid anything extra. We're not sharing in that benefit even though it's us who make it possible. It isn't fair."

They arrived at the coffee machine, which was positioned on a table littered with used cups, plastic spoons, spilled sugar, and soiled napkins.

"Look at this," Ralph huffed. "The guy is a millionaire and we have to get our coffee from a pig trough."

At his desk fifteen minutes later, Smith tried to forget about what Ralph had told him. The guy was a notorious complainer, always whining about some minor injustice, while at the same time hustling to sell Phillies tickets, among other things. Mark Wexler himself had to trudge up the stairs, and his office was on the twelfth floor. If the boss was making a few extra dollars because of the reduced energy use, at least he had to go the distance on his own two feet.

Although still unsettled about Timmy, Smith tried to focus on his work. He told himself to make the most of the first hour of the day. He couldn't put in his request for a time off until the Human Resources Department opened at ten o'clock anyway. He switched on his computer, watched the screen come alive, and mulled over where he had left off on Friday.

Mark Wexler had recruited Smith directly from Drexel University. Back then, Wexler Associates was growing, building its business upon the revitalization of Philadelphia's waterfront. The channel leading from the Atlantic Ocean, up the Delaware Bay and River, all the way to the city itself, had been deepened. This reality required the oil refineries, chemical plants, and commercial wharves to rebuild their facilities to accommodate deeper draft ships. Wexler put together a team of specialists, among them Robert Smith, to design and supervise these projects. Those had been heady days, filled with late nights, early mornings, and site visits aboard boats, barges, and even helicopters.

Not anymore. It wasn't Mr. Wexler's fault the company contracted over the past few years. There just wasn't the volume of work that there had been. If anything, he kept the company afloat by landing lucrative contracts for government-funded projects, such as the one on which Smith currently toiled.

His computer screen displayed a color-coded topographical map of the thirty-acre swath at Central West. This wasn't the first time a beautiful new complex was to rise on the site. The same thing had been promised a half dozen times over the preceding decades. Now, however, the President himself said that projects like this were needed to jump-start the economy, to keep good people in good-paying jobs, as well as to meet the demand for critical services to the less fortunate. Congress agreed. Thus, the project included several residential towers to accommodate people who couldn't afford the rising cost of a home within the city limits.

The foundations for these towers were Smith's biggest challenge. Over the millennia, receding glaciers churned up the earth, alternately leaving behind boulders and fine silt. Central West was mostly silt, and building anything atop it was like standing in mud. Eventually you sank to the bottom, or worse, you fell over. There were solutions, none of which were cheap.

As he contemplated the possibilities, Smith stole glances at his cell phone. Hannah should have called him by now, but there was neither a voice mail nor a text message indicated on his screen. He decided against calling; she would only be annoyed by his nagging.

Just before ten, Smith left his desk for Human Resources. What once occupied a small corner of the second floor currently spanned the building. A row of teller windows separated the department from waiting employees, who all looked as if they'd been in line for hours. Smith hadn't expected any delay here. He wished that he'd switched off his computer instead of just the monitor. If an Energy Auditor discovered he was away for more than fifteen minutes without shutting down his desk equipment, he might receive an official reprimand, or worse, a fine.

He glanced at his watch, noted that he'd only been standing there a few minutes, and figured it wouldn't hurt to jog back upstairs to power things down. Just as he turned to leave the room he saw Henny Geerman coming in bearing a stack of binders. Mrs. Geerman had been the payroll clerk who introduced Smith to the world of Wexler Associates. She completed the paperwork, took his photo for his I.D. badge, even kissed him on the cheek when he told her that Mr. Wexler had made him an offer.

"A sweet offer it is," she'd said as she finished his payroll documents. She went on to become the head of the department.

Smith stepped up to her with his arms out to help with the binders. She happily surrendered half of them with a puff.

"Leave it to a foundation guy to carry the load," she said. "How are you these days?"

"Mostly good."

"Must be something wrong if you're here. We'll have to update your I.D. while we're at it. That thing is a relic."

Smith reflexively looked at his badge. It showed a much younger man.

"Come to my office. If you get stuck in this line you'll be here all day."

They passed through a security door, deep into the human resources department, where Geerman took a seat behind her desk in a private office. Smith couldn't help but marvel at this space given that no one other than the most senior members of the firm had their own offices anymore.

Geerman picked up on Smith's fascination. She said, "We deal with personal information here. That's why we get our own offices."

"I used to have one," Smith said with a nod. "Conservation rules did away with it."

Geerman sighed. "That's a shame. Sometimes you need to be alone with your thoughts, especially if you're a team leader. A bunch of psychologists were in here wanting to do a research project on the subject, but they never finalized the thing. Probably lost their funding."

"These aren't the best of times," Smith commented.

Geerman found places for each of the binders then asked, "How can I help you today, Bob?"

"I need a day off," he answered, "for a medical situation."

"My gosh! Here we are chatting. You should have said something right away. Let's get this done."

Smith felt a swell of relief in his chest. At the same time, his comfort was diminished by a tinge of guilt at having circumvented the line. Cutting ahead was not the act of a leader. What would he say if Timmy did it?

"It's my son," he said quietly. "I need to get a second opinion."

"Oh my."

"I hope the second opinion finds something else," Smith said. "Tomorrow, I'd like to go to my Health Administration District Office for an approval. Then I'll need another day off to take him to the specialist."

Using her computer, Geerman accessed Smith's personnel file. She scanned several different screens then clucked her tongue. "Bob," she said softly, "you have to come see me more often."

"What do you mean?"

"You missed the deadline to convert your vacation days."

"I don't understand," Smith said.

"Didn't you get the email? The one that said vacation time is no longer cumulative? It's a Federal Mandate, part of the Wage Stabilization and Equalization Act."

Smith never paid attention to the emails from Human Resources. They were always about the company picnic or an update on the sexual harassment policy. As for his vacation days, he had been accumulating them to take Timmy to see the country's natural wonders, Civil War battlefields, and major cities. Naturally, these journeys depended on his ability to secure the gasoline, but Smith was working on a solution to that, too.

"Gosh," Geerman said next. "You're going to have to use them or lose them by the end of the year."

By Smith's own estimation, he had at least ten weeks saved. How was he going to use that many days before the end of the year when Central West was kicking off? However that issue resolved itself, he needed a couple free days to take care of Timmy. The Universal Coverage Manual explicitly stated that he was entitled, by law, to days off for medical emergencies, and those days were to be paid leave, not vacation days.

"Put me down for tomorrow with a second day pending," he said to Geerman.

"Sure, Bob, I'm doing that right now." Her hands danced over the keys before she pulled them back to her lap. "Let me have your badge again," she said. "I have to cross check something."

Smith unclipped his I.D., handed it to Geerman, and leaned back in his chair. The wall clock indicated he'd been away from his desk for ten minutes. He confirmed the time on his watch and shifted forward to see what his host was doing.

"I suppose you can take tomorrow off without penalty," Geerman said, "but it'll have to be unpaid, one of your personal days."

"Unpaid?" Smith blurted. "The Universal Coverage Manual says that I can have up to six months off, with pay, for a medical emergency. I'm only asking for two days!"

Geerman gave him a friendly smile. She was used to people more adamant and difficult than Robert Smith. "You are Bob, except that your internal file has you listed on a CGP. CGP's are exempt from the regulations you might have read in the UCM."

"CGP? What's that?"

She truly thought he was joking, and Geerman paused for the punchline. When it didn't come, she realized that Smith was a goal-oriented guy who only dealt with the mission at hand.

"A Critical Government Project," she said ticking off the letters with the fingers of her left hand. "I'm guessing that the government exempted itself from the UCM regulations to keep military and other important personnel on the job in times of crisis."

"I'm getting ready to oversee the site prep crew at Central West. We're not building a nuclear missile silo," Smith explained. "Even if I did meet the President last week."

"You did?" Geerman said pleasantly. "I'm impressed."

Frustrated, Smith wiped the corners of his mouth and took a deep breath. "Henny," he said, "I'm taking off tomorrow. I need to get Timmy's second opinion in the works."

"I understand. Just so you know, it'll be without pay. That Wage Stabilization and Equalization Act has real teeth to it. We're subject to a quarterly audit and if we show any breech of fairness there is a huge fine."

Smith nodded. "I get it. I can't even use one of my vacation days that are about to evaporate?"

"Maybe," she answered. "You'd have to get approval."

"You're in charge of the department," he said hopefully.

"CGP approvals have to come from Mr. Wexler. Do you want me to ask him?"

The last thing Smith wanted was to bring the matter before Mr. Wexler, who was less congenial when not in the presence of high-ranking officials. Wexler was a by-the-book type who quoted chapter and verse from regulations and manuals as if he had a photographic memory. For all Smith knew, the man might be so endowed.

"Thanks, Henny. Please see what you can do about extending my vacation time to next year. I'd like to take Timmy on some trips then."

Smith got to his feet, listening half-heartedly to Geerman's platitudes and best wishes for Timmy health.

He trudged up the stairs, struggling with the bad news Geerman had given him. Losing a day's pay would dent his budget. There would be a second one, too, unless he could work it out with Hannah to take Timmy to the doctor. Although he understood the logic of the government's rules, Smith wasn't happy about the way they were applied. His was not a job on which the country's security depended. He wasn't tending to a nuclear reactor or guarding convicted felons or managing air traffic control. His team could easily handle their duties without him for a week, let alone a day, and when it came time to actually build Central West, there would be inevitable delays caused by weather, labor strikes, and supply shortages.

He walked with his head down, grumbling to himself, re-calculating his family's budget. He arrived at his cube to find Ralph occupying the space.

Surprised, Smith asked, "What are you doing here?"

"Saving your ass," Ralph replied indignantly. "Next time you go for a waltz be sure to shut down your machine."

"The screen was off."

"Yeah, like any Energy Auditor wouldn't hear that cooling fan whizzing away. They clip the whole team when the leader breaks the rules."

"I know," Smith offered humbly. "Sorry."

"No sweat, boss. I'm looking out for all of us. By the way, you need any tickets to the Phillies? I got a couple of pairs. Great seats. You and Timmy could be sitting behind home plate, close enough to be the umpire."

The cheering, sugary soft drinks, and greasy food were the last things Timmy needed. Smith declined the offer and rolled his chair into position.

"I got a line on a few gas vouchers, too," Ralph persisted. "Up to twelve gallons if you know how to work it."

"No thanks," Smith said. "Let's get to work."

ALL CLIENTS WILL BE ASSIGNED A NUMBER.

CHAPTER
FOUR

BITTER ABOUT HIS SITUATION, Smith told none of his junior team members that he wouldn't be at work the next day. No one needed to know, except for Josh. Smith waited to tell him until they were nearly home.

"We're on hold until the test boring results come in," Josh said upon hearing Smith's news. "Not much will be going on."

"Keep an eye on Ralph," Smith warned. "Make sure he calls about those borings."

"Will do," Josh nodded.

"I don't know about those Phillies tickets he sells either. There's a lottery held for the best seats and how could he win it so often?"

"I have no idea," Josh admitted, adding as he exited the pickup, "I hope everything goes well for you tomorrow."

Of all the houses in Cliffwood, Smith knew that his was the best. It had been one of the models. For the trouble of prospective buyers traipsing through it, Smith had received a ten-percent discount on the asking price of similar, unviewed homes. It also featured many upgrades at no additional charge such as the extra wide garage, custom closets, hardwood floors, and so forth. Not wanting to be a braggart, he never mentioned these things to people. Visitors were awed upon entering the house and discovering its many amenities.

"This is nice," they would say. "Very nice."

The house was a source of pride for him, a quiet, internal, perhaps selfish delight. After two weeks living within its walls he couldn't remember how he survived a dingy apartment that had truly been a prison: square rooms, hardly any natural light, and too many shared spaces with other tenants.

The only problem with Smith's suburban masterpiece was the transportation. Well, that and the taxes, both of which continued to rise. The mortgage and real estate taxes consumed Hannah's entire salary. Keeping their vehicles on the road and the rest of their necessities left him with little cash to set aside.

Lately, Smith considered getting a second job to finance Timmy's education. He was willing to do whatever he had to for his son's future, but second jobs weren't available in the suburbs. Even the convenience stores were disappearing, not that this was his preferred alternative. It was simply that year by year, things were migrating toward the city. He couldn't help but wonder if he should follow some of his neighbors and make the move himself.

Then again, if the President had his way, college would be just like high school, free to everyone who qualified. All his fret-

ting over the house, the price of gas, and Timmy's baseball scholarship might be for nothing.

"I thought you'd had a stroke," Hannah said as Smith came
through the door. "You were standing out there, staring like a
lost sheep."

"I'm alright," Smith lied, though he wasn't in the mood to
talk.

"You want to hear some good news?" she prompted.

"If it's free."

"It's better than free."

Raising his eyebrows, Smith asked, "Are you sure?"

She led him to the dining room table where a number of
official forms lay scattered. Hannah's block printing occupied
some of the boxes.

"It pays to ask," Hannah began. "I met with the principal at
Timmy's school."

"What about the nurse?" Smith interrupted.

"Sure. I spoke to her, too. First, let me tell you what the principal told me. Because of Timmy's condition, we can apply for a
special M Fuel Supplement Card available only to people with
approved medical conditions. I think Timmy's is on the list."

A moment passed while Smith registered what this meant.
"Really?"

"I'm almost done with the application. When this is approved, Timmy won't have to ride the bus. I'll take him to school
and pick him up every day."

"But you're not finished until four."

"That's what the other application is all about," Hannah explained.

"The other application?"

"Yeah. The one I did online for us to become Certified Caregivers."

"We're his parents," Smith scoffed. "What more certification do we need?"

"Without the certification process, non-traditional families would be excluded," Hannah explained. "The point is, I'll be allowed to leave work early. We'll qualify for the M Fuel Card and have the gas to take Timmy back and forth to school and his doctor appointments."

"We'll still have to pay ten dollars a gallon for it," Smith moaned.

Hannah dropped her pen on the table. She said, "Be happy, Bob. Don't ruin a perfectly good evening, okay?"

That wasn't his intention. He'd just been calculating the family's cost of living and he'd done the math in light of Henny Geerman's bad news. To that he might have subtracted the amount of Hannah's certain pay cut when she started leaving work an hour and a half early to tote their son both ways to school. Although, according to the UCM, her pay couldn't be cut. He was glad to have the extra gasoline, even if it would be a stretch to pay for it.

Instead of reminding Hannah of these facts, he said, "I'm taking off tomorrow to get the second opinion approval."

"Good," his wife acknowledged without looking at him.

Despite the tension in the air, Smith felt his stomach rumble. He'd grown up on hot suppers cooked by his mother and looked forward to them. With rare exception it was the three of them around the table. His father always washed his hands but never managed to cleanse the grease from his cracked skin. Sometimes he'd miss a smudge on his forehead and Smith's mother would take a napkin from the table and wipe it off. These moments Smith remembered fondly, wishing he shared more of them with Hannah. Too often she ate her supper in front of the TV while he and Timmy foraged for themselves.

To boost his spirits and capture a bit of nostalgia, he said, "Let me help you with supper, honey."

They decided to make veggie burgers complete with all the trimmings. It was an indoor cookout, made all the more fun by a small fire on the stove and ensuing smoke in the kitchen. Timmy, who had been in a funk when they started, began to have fun at the table. He hung onions from his mouth like Dracula fangs and added ketchup to prove the Dark Prince had taken a bite from some innocent's neck.

Father and son settled into the living room where they watched *On The Prowl*, a crime series featuring a character named Detective Ted Elroy. After the bad guy had been caught they retired for the night.

"Mom says I'm not going to be on the bus anymore," Timmy said as he climbed into bed.

"We'll see," Smith replied. "I'm going to visit some people tomorrow. They'll get you straightened out."

"My friends are all on the bus, dad. They'll forget about me if I'm not there."

"Nobody's going to forget you, Timmy. You're the best player on the team."

"I am," Timmy said with pride.

"Remember what we talked about yesterday?"

"Yeah."

"It's just for a little while. Once we get you fixed up, you'll be trying out for the Phillies."

"First, I'm taking the Media Moguls to the regional championship, dad."

"That's a good plan, son," Smith finished.

◆• •◆• •◆•

Health Administration District Office Number 117 had all the charm of a soggy cardboard box. Streaks of rust stained the exterior of the building, the cause of which Bob Smith could not imagine. The reflective coating peeled from the corner of every window. Had there not been a sign beside the entrance, Smith might have thought he'd come to the wrong place. But there it was, standing like a tombstone among patches of weeds, announcing to employees and visitors alike that they were, in fact, at their intended destination.

Despite the shabby look of the building, Smith felt remarkably upbeat. It appeared that he was the first one to arrive, surely a good sign. Plus, he was organized. A neat folder contained Timmy's paperwork from the hospital. He brought a pair of fresh pens and a pad of paper to take notes. He was prepared and ready to navigate the system, the one he and Hannah had rallied for in college. How complicated could it be?

Inside the building was hardly better than outside. A surly guard asked Smith what he was doing there an hour before any of the offices opened.

"I thought I'd get here early," Smith explained. "I'm hoping to get back to work later this morning."

The guard smirked, pointed to a placard of rules, the first of which read: ALL CLIENTS WILL BE ASSIGNED A NUMBER.

"Good," Smith said. "I suppose I'll be number one."

This provoked the guard into a fit of laughter. Not getting the joke, Smith stood there with a slack grin on his face.

"The numbers don't go out for another half hour. You can

wait outside until then."

"I can't wait in here?"

"Against regulations," the guard answered.

Smith retreated to his pickup where he promptly scrolled through the radio dial. He settled on the all-news station. While the daily headlines were read, he saw the guard come out of the building and then rummage around in the weeds about ten feet from the door. After a few seconds the guard stood up, shrugged, and walked back inside. Smith thought this was odd, but the radio announcer caught his attention with a report that unemployment for the month had dropped one tenth of one percent.

"The President's spokesperson issued a statement that the increase in employment is proof the administration's stimulus program is working. In sports, Derek Jackson shows he's worth his multi-million dollar contract by hitting two home runs against ..."

By the end of the first commercial break, Smith noted that several vehicles had entered the lot. He decided to go back to the entrance in case a line had formed there. His instincts were right. He ambled up to the last person who had brought her own folding chair.

"Is it like this all the time?"

The woman looked up at him and replied, "Must be your first visit."

"It is," Smith confirmed.

"If you got a major problem, I suggest you get a seat like this one," she said. "My son used to take it camping with him. Folds up to nothing and is light as a leaf."

From an engineering standpoint, Smith appreciated the good design of the chair. He also remembered waiting in line like this for concert tickets.

"Yeah, I got a couple plugged arteries, a bad knee, a slipped disc, L5-S1, and without this thing, I'd probably be lying on the ground."

"I'm sorry to hear that."

"So am I," she said. "Been out of work for two years now. Spend half my time right here and the other half chasing down the appointments they give me."

The person in line ahead of her, an elderly woman with a walker glared back at the one who was speaking loud enough to be heard across the street.

"You look pretty solid," she was saying to Smith. "What brings you here?"

"I'm fine," Smith replied. "My son needs a second opinion."

"Oh. That's too bad."

More people arrived, some with chairs, others with the same look on their face as Smith: What's this line all about? He took comfort in his position, fifth from the door. He couldn't help but feel sorry for those behind him.

Just before nine another security guard showed up. He wore a white hat, shoes that gleamed, and a name tag which identified him as "RIESER." His presence caused a stir among several in the line. He went inside for a few minutes then returned to address the crowd, all of whom were now on their feet. He carried a roll of tickets in one hand and a note card in the other.

"Russo, Paulson, Bridge, Klein, Tennant!" hollered Rieser.

The lady beside Smith bolted from the line to be the first up to Rieser. He tore the first ticket off the roll and handed it to her. Smith thought she was pretty spry for a woman with a bad knee, a slipped disc, and plugged arteries.

When those tickets had been given out, Rieser called more names. He repeated the process six times, after which he stuffed the note card into his back pocket.

"No litter. No arguments. No blocking the entrance. No trouble whatsoever or you'll be remanded to custody," he said in a powerful voice. "Is that understood?"

No one answered.

"Good."

When Rieser was out of earshot, Smith heard a nearby voice say, "This is criminal. No?"

"Mr. Fetterman," Smith said, acknowledging one of Timmy's biggest fans and another of his father's former regulars. Fetterman never missed a Moguls game. He stood along the outfield wall, hoisting his arms in the air with each hit.

"You need a liver biopsy like me?" Mr. Fetterman asked.

"No, I'm getting an approval for a second opinion." He didn't mention Timmy so as not to upset a fan.

"You'll have that before lunch," Fetterman was saying. "I'll be lucky if I don't expire before I get things straightened out."

Seeing that thirty people were now in front of him, Smith had his doubts about leaving before noon.

"Next time you just slip Rieser's buddy something and you'll be in the first batch. In and out of here in an hour or less."

"Are you serious?" Smith asked.

Fetterman shrugged his sagging shoulders. "Get here early and give a few shekels to that other uniform. I can't remember his name. He passes it on to Rieser along with your name and you've got your number."

"You mean those people bribed the guards?"

"Sure they did, and you'll be smart if you call them security officers and not guards."

Incensed, Smith felt his face flush at how an orderly and fair system had been so easily corrupted. Hadn't he felt uneasy about cutting the line yesterday at Human Resources? Yet, these feck-less people thought nothing of it. They were willing to buy a spot in lieu of waiting.

"Mind your temper," Fetterman warned. "Rieser can send you packing for nothing more than a dirty look. I've seen it happen."

His earlier enthusiasm gone, Smith stared into space, occasionally shuffling forward when someone ahead took their turn.

His number, given to him by Rieser, was thirty-seven. Smith held the ticket for two and a half hours before the display at the head of the room indicated his turn had finally come. A hundred and fifty minutes of waiting gave him ample time to organize his thoughts as well as to rehearse what he wanted to say to whomever it was he would meet. There was no way he was going to stand by in the face of the crudest forms of corruption. This wasn't the Bureau of Motor Vehicles; this was about health-care, people's lives were affected. If the person didn't take him seriously then he would start complaining to the next one up the ladder until someone listened and did something. Squeaky wheels get the oil, he reminded himself.

Just as he got to the front of the room he made eye contact with Mr. Fetterman. The gent put a finger over his lips and blew softly.

"Shhhhhh."

Smith couldn't help but nod his head. He stowed his complaint for later, after Timmy was taken care of. Maybe he would videotape these so-called security men committing their petty crimes. He would be a hero instead of a chump. He might even get extra gas rations as a reward, or season tickets for the Phillies.

All the waiting paid off in that Smith got what he wanted: an authorization to obtain a second opinion. Although, he wasn't completely satisfied. As the friendly Care Administration Specialist explained to him, the details of the appointment would be sent in the mail. Exactly when, the specialist couldn't say, but she assured him the case would be reviewed quickly.

"There have been a lot of problems at Media General lately, but don't worry. They'll get straightened out eventually," she finished. "We'll send you an email so you don't have to wait for the hard copy in the regular mail."

He was glad to hear that, especially because the United States Postal Service only delivered three times per week in the suburbs.

Leaving the parking lot, he cringed at the ugly building behind him. The sight in his rearview mirror did nothing to relieve his worries. He desperately wanted to pile Timmy into the truck and take him to the first heart specialist he could find. The trouble was that the doctor wouldn't see him. Not only were all the appointments booked, it was against the rules. The Care Administration Specialist explained this and read several more rules from a laminated card. Paying for a spot in line was also against the rules, Smith thought, but no one was doing anything about that.

He shook his head in disgust and drove on.

He initially headed for work. It was only a few minutes past one o'clock, and several hours of analysis was exactly what Central West needed. Then he remembered that he wasn't getting paid for the day. Why should he waste the gas driving to a payless job? If Timmy wasn't in school he would have taken him for a brief ride through the nearby countryside. In the end, Smith decided to drive to his father's old service station.

He almost missed it, stopping a few dozen yards beyond the edge of the property. Given his lack of fuel, not to mention shortage of time, Smith had not been here in years. The gas station had cornered the intersection of two rural routes, one that led southeast toward Media, the other tracing a line generally west toward Lancaster.

Smith grew up in a comfortable house a mile away, the son of a man who'd been a sergeant in the United States Army and a woman who worked part time in a bakery. He went off to college a single man, eager to experience that rite of passage without the baggage of a steady girlfriend. Later in his education, he met Hannah, who quickly became his sole female companion, much to the disappointment of girls he previously dated.

Standing in the weed-strewn lot that once contained his father's station, Smith reflected on the days when he worked here. From an early age, he knew he wouldn't be following in his father's footsteps. Still, he enjoyed his time here. There were regular customers, people who watched him grow up, who spoke highly of his father's mechanical skill. At Christmas they would give him small treats. When they learned of his acceptance to college, there were universal congratulations. He almost felt guilty about leaving the fold. At the same time, he recognized that these customers wanted him to move on with his life. It was their patronage of his father's business that made his life possible.

"They pay the bills, not me," his father said. "Don't ever forget that."

Smith didn't forget. He infused this sensibility into his work ethic at Wexler Associates.

His father's garage had three bays, an attached office, and two islands with pumps. Between those pumps was a tall stool, which was rarely used.

"If I catch you sitting on your butt instead of doing something for a customer, I'll fire you," his father told every new hire.

Only federally licensed Fuel Depots dispensed gasoline now. Each one had an official monitor with his own second floor office, from which he watched the goings-on closer than Smith's father ever had. The larger ones had a Federal Energy Police Station on site, ready to respond in the event of a robbery or other incident. The people who worked the pumps where not referred to as gas jockeys but rather Pee-Tee's, which was short for Petroleum Product Transfer Specialist.

Standing atop the concrete pad that formed the base of the missing pumps, Smith smiled at having been a part-time gas jockey. He figured he'd get a written reprimand from someone in Henny Geerman's department if he used the term inside the Wexler Building. Whatever the case, the attendants, including Smith, quickly learned the regulars' names, including Mr. Hilti who drove a Ford Crown Victoria and his cousin, Gary Semanoff, whose Buick LeSabre never seemed to get dirty. Then there were the Penner sisters whose father bought them matching Chevrolet Camaros. How could he forget Mr. Fetterman's land yacht, a lengthy Cadillac Sedan DeVille, or Doctor Ben's new pickups!

Shortly after the cancer diagnosis, Smith's father closed up, much to the surprise and dismay of his customers. There was never the issue of Smith operating the business. He was on his way up the ladder at Wexler Associates, earning a healthy salary, managing a few journeymen of his own. What did he want with a gas station that required endless supervision and provided less money than his regular job?

Smith sold his inheritance quick, and therefore cheap, but the money was portable whereas the property was not. He spent it on a number of things, many of which he could not remember. He did recall the smell of the garage, a combination of sweet grease and the acrid diesel fuel in which his father cleaned tools. There was also the hint of peanuts, his father's favorite snack. A giant can of them sat on the counter for workers and customers alike.

There had been a roadside inn on the other corner. Over the years it served every purpose imaginable from a restaurant, to a veterinary clinic, to a warehouse. It had been demolished, the stone foundation removed, and a layer of grass planted atop the plot. Farther down the road, a strip of stores no longer offered video rentals, a quick pizza, or office supplies. Bit by bit the landscape was returning to the rural countryside it had been in the eighteenth century. As the price of transportation increased, people migrated toward towns and cities, taking their business with them.

I'm lucky to have sold the station when I did, Smith thought.

There were a few holdouts, mostly people with an interest in agriculture or forestry. Some wealthy individuals advertised their desire to purchase real estate. A government program to relieve distressed mortgage holders ceased when it became oversubscribed. Banks with large real estate portfolios failed, their assets ending up as government holdings that were sometimes auctioned off or else used to expand state parks and game lands.

While he rambled down the empty lane, not a vehicle passed by. During his father's tenure, such a phenomenon wouldn't have happened except for the latest hours of the night. Even then, a lone State Policeman, truck driver, or philanderer would be rolling along this stretch of road. Smith wondered if he missed the end of the world, if he was caught in some sort of time warp. Not that the country wasn't trying. The President, and Congress for that matter, worked tirelessly on elaborate stimulus programs designed to create jobs and spur economic growth. Smith supported these efforts wholeheartedly as his own job was dependent upon one. He knew that sometimes the government had to takeover when the private sector simply couldn't do enough to invigorate the country, and according to the news report, unemployment had fallen and things were starting to turn around.

He drove his truck toward Media. Actually, he coasted most of the distance, thankful that he still had the money and fuel ration to drive his own vehicle. He felt entitled to these, which given his position as a team leader were more necessity than luxury. What if a meeting was held at a job site? What if a storm caused the Delaware River to flood and they needed him to inspect the stability of the bridge piers? These were not remote possibilities but rather likely occurrences.

He didn't mind riding the FART. Its cars weren't the best and delays plagued the system, but Smith believed in the concept of mass transit. It was more efficient than personal vehicles and thereby caused less pollution. In its present form it needed some tweaking, but every form of technology evolved over time. Smith was convinced suburban transit would do the same and consequently restore the appeal of semi-rural living.

In contrast, Philadelphia's Subway and Elevated Rail system had never been better. Renamed the Central Transport Authority, or CTA, it featured new lines linking every part of the city. Beautiful stations replaced the dreary stops of the past. Unfortunately, where the subway terminated, there ended this level of service. As it was, passengers transferring between the FART and CTA systems had to walk six blocks to make the connection. Whenever this fact came up in conversation, Smith shook his head and commented, "They're coming. They're coming," referring to the integrated stations that would allow direct transfers.

In the center of Media, Smith decided to do something

special for Timmy, the cost be damned. He had credit cards, didn't he? Leaving his truck, he walked briskly along Baltimore Avenue, turning north on Edgemont, and continuing to Third Street. There he was pleased to discover the shop to which his father had taken him thirty years ago was still open.

"ROBERT!"

Smith snapped his head around, taking his eyes off Timmy for just a second. He saw Hannah marching directly toward him, her arms swinging. A lovely woman when she wasn't angry, Hannah could be downright ugly when provoked. At the moment, her face displayed the kind of rage that Smith had seen only a few times in their marriage.

"What are you doing?" Hannah demanded. She was less than ten feet away and had not decreased the volume of her voice a single decibel.

For the life of him, Smith couldn't figure out what he'd done wrong. He kept Timmy's surprise a secret through supper and for an hour afterward. By that time, he was eager to see the boy smile. It was Timmy's last day riding the bus, something that left him moping about the house. Smith took him into the garage, hoisted the brand new bicycle he'd bought earlier in the afternoon out of the back of his pickup, and presented it to his son. Timmy's excitement was nothing compared to the joy Smith felt at the sight of his son's grin.

"Remember not to overexert yourself," Smith warned. "Just coast around the block."

"Okay, dad," Timmy beamed as he rolled out of the garage.

Now Hannah was standing at Smith's side, with her hands on her hips. "Where is your brain?" she asked.

Smith stole a glance at Timmy then turned to face his wife.

"It's right here," he said.

"After what the nurse told us, you thought it was a good idea to buy Timmy a bicycle?"

"I told him to take it easy. Just coast around on it."

"And you think he'll listen?" Hannah retorted.

This angered Smith more than his wife's lack of appreciation for what he'd done to lift Timmy's spirits. "He's a good boy," Smith reminded her.

"TIMMY!" Hannah yelled.

Timmy skidded to a stop then turned slowly toward his parents.

"Let him go," Smith said.

"For someone who was worried enough to take a day off of work to get a second opinion, you seem not to care at all about what the nurse said."

After taking a second to collect his thoughts, Smith said, "I've been thinking about that. We never actually spoke to the doctor."

"He works in the emergency room, Bob. He doesn't have time to hang out for a chat."

"He should have spoken to us directly."

"I think the nurse did a thorough job of explaining the situation. You also have the Primary Cardiac Care booklet or whatever it is."

Holding his ground, Smith said, "I'm going to check through the Universal Coverage Manual to see what the rules are. I think we're entitled to speak with the doctor."

Hannah shook her head. "What if there were people waiting for him? Better yet, what if you were lying on the table bleeding from a car crash or something? Would you want him to have a bull session with some other Bob Smith?"

"We're entitled to the same care as anyone else," Smith said pedantically. "I suspect there may be another reason why he didn't want to talk to us."

"And what might that be detective?"

"Maybe he didn't speak English," Smith said offhandedly.

Hannah shoved him hard with both hands and stomped away.

"What was that for?" Smith hollered as he recovered his balance. He pursued her across the lawn, not catching up until they reached the kitchen door.

Turning to face her husband, Hannah said quietly, "What's gotten into you, Bob?"

"Gotten into me?" he replied indignantly.

Keeping her tone even and her face impassive, Hannah answered, "That was the question, but let me ask another one. Do you remember the things we did in college?"

"In college? What are you talking about?"

"We're talking about you, Bob, and the tolerant guy you are, or maybe the intolerant guy you're becoming. Back in college, you weren't one of those white guys from the suburbs who stuck to his own kind. You weren't afraid to cross those invisible boundaries less enlightened people create."

Smith couldn't discern whether it was shame or embarrassment or something else that made his face flush. Hannah clarified for him.

She said, "It's okay to be angry when confronted with your intolerance."

To this point, Smith hadn't been angry, but now he understood that Hannah interpreted his remark about the doctor not speaking English as an assault on the man's race. Nothing could be further from the truth. From what few words the doctor had spoken how could anyone tell the slightest thing about him? As for his complexion, he might have been from India, Spain, Italy, anywhere in South America, or around the corner. And what difference did that make? Smith wanted to talk about his son's heart, not about anyone's heritage.

"If you want to talk about what we did in college, you'll remember I was a founding member of the Committee to Diversify Admissions," Smith explained.

"Yes, you were," Hannah agreed.

"And you're accusing me of being a bigot?"

"It's probably a latent thing, like a suppressed habit, something learned from your father that surfaces during times of stress."

"I resent that," Smith said with more force than he intended.

She smiled cautiously then replied, "It's a natural reaction. Both of us are upset about Timmy's condition. I'm dealing with it. You're reacting badly. You lash out against a doctor that issued a diagnosis you can't accept. You buy Timmy a bicycle as a further act of denial. You're ignoring reality every step of the way. It's the first phase of the coping process, but you have to move on."

Although her explanation made too much sense for him to deny, Smith refused to acquiesce. "Asking a doctor to justify his conclusions is nothing less than what I have to do every day. I happen to speak English, so it's not too much to ask that he do the same."

Hannah dropped her smile and shifted on her feet. "For a moment let's say you're right. Let's say that we only let doctors practice medicine if they speak the King's English. Do you know where that would leave us?"

Sensing a trap, Smith glanced at his shoes instead of opening his mouth.

"If you'd watch the news once in a while you'd know that there is a shortage of doctors in this country, Bob. Enrollment at domestic medical schools has been falling for years. Therefore, it's no surprise that the doctors you're going to meet may not speak English as well as you and I. It's not their fault. It's our fault. We aren't doing enough on our side of the oceans. We have to reach out to other places where people understand that medicine is about caring for people instead of getting rich. That's why the doctor who examined Timmy looks and speaks the way he does. He's a good Samaritan in the selfish world of an America that still doesn't get it."

Smith let her have the point. He might have overreacted. It was the first time since he'd become a father that Timmy had anything worse than the flu. Simultaneously, he wondered why his son's heart problem hadn't been detected during his annual school physical or one of the exams before baseball season.

Hannah, on the other hand, wasn't finished. She said, "Thanks to that doctor, whom you don't think very much of, Timmy was treated quickly and professionally. If it wasn't for Universal Coverage, who knows what might have happened?"

Thoroughly beaten, Smith could do nothing but look away. Out of the corner of his eye, he saw Timmy walking his bike up the driveway. The boy disappeared into the garage. A moment later, the automatic door closed with a hum.

CHAPTER
FIVE

DURING HIS COLLEGE YEARS, Bob Smith joined a student sit-in at Drexel, traveled to D.C. to walk twenty-five times around the Capitol Building in an organized protest, and stuffed literally thousands of fliers in mailboxes and under doors all in support of healthcare for every American. Healthcare, he believed then and still believed now, was a right, something every person deserved regardless of their social status. The best possible care was to be delivered in a prompt and efficient manner. The wealthy always had this luxury, which, to the young Smith's way of thinking, was a horrible injustice. Why should someone be denied care just because they didn't have the money? Didn't the Declaration of Independence mention that all men were created equal? The

Universal Healthcare and Medical Assistance Act, Universal Coverage for short, affirmed that they were and was specifically designed to put an end to inequalities in an area of American society that desperately needed a bit of leveling.

With all that in mind, Smith simmered over Hannah's accusation. How could he be as she described him when he'd done so much to the contrary? Considering that his father's platoon was a mixed group of various races, how could she say that he was a racist? "Bullets don't know the color of your skin," his father had once said. "You fight together and win, or you die alone in defeat." These words Smith carried with him to those sit-ins and protests, to the voting booth, and to every job he worked.

He reviewed these facts in the days after their argument. If only he'd thought of them sooner, he might have better defended himself. No matter, the authorization for Timmy's second opinion had yet to come via regular or electronic means, which aggravated him that much more. The people he voted for those years ago crafted definitive legislation to reach poorly served geographic areas, to reduce the cost of necessary drugs, and to construct new clinics across the country. Thanks to their diligent pursuit of the stated goals, Smith himself worked on the foundation for a brand new medical facility to be built at Central West.

Still, he waited nearly a week with no response from the HAO. This was not how it was supposed to be, and he was getting ready to do something about it. He couldn't specify what he was going to do, not exactly, but he wanted to show Hannah he was capable of doing it without offending anybody.

Sitting at his desk, he was just putting the finishing touches on a report about possible cost increases at Central West when the public address system chimed three times.

"Please back up your data," an elegant female voice announced from ceiling-mounted speakers.

A collective groan rose from the people working in their cubes.

"Energy conservation will begin in five minutes," the voice continued. "Information integrity is your responsibility. Please back up your data."

In a burst of anger, Smith pounded his fist on his desk. His notebook leapt into the air along with his pencils, cell phone, and empty coffee cup. He needed no more than ten minutes to finish his work, but now something as simple as a rudimentary report was interrupted by an arbitrarily imposed Energy Conservation Event. Any electrical engineer worth half a week's pay could design a system to stagger the cut-off for individual workstations. As it was, Smith was stuck with the generic arrangement that darkened the entire building.

Any other day this would not have been a big deal, but there was the looming circumstance of not receiving the authorization for a second opinion, something that caused him to lose a fair amount of sleep. So far, Timmy was doing fine aside of being sullen about not riding the bus with his pals.

Typing as fast as he could, Smith failed to keep up with the voice on the PA that reminded him, "Two minutes until energy conservation begins. Data backup should be complete at this time. Lost data may result in lost wages. Back up your data now."

He surrendered to the faceless decree, saving his file in the nick of time and smacking the off switch for his monitor before the electricity stopped flowing. Just the same, his frustration did not abate. He glanced at his cell phone, which had the capability of accessing his email account. There were no messages.

Resisting the urge to scream, he pulled a folded piece of

paper from his hip pocket and smoothed it over his desk blotter. He punched the number written there into his cell phone. A second later he relaxed as the connection went through. Then a recorded voice dashed his hopes.

"Health Administration District Office Number 117 is currently closed as part of the national energy management effort. Thank you for doing your part to arrest global warming and improve energy security for the nation. Goodbye."

If the phone hadn't cost him hundreds of dollars he would have thrown it across the room. As it was, he couldn't afford to replace it, and he wasn't a violent man by nature. In fact, he was disappointed in his own thoughts and behavior. For all he knew, there might be a perfectly legitimate reason for the delay in the second opinion. As far as energy conservation was concerned, he agreed with that, too. Global warming had the potential to ruin the planet for the very son he wanted so much to be cured. Everyone had to do their part, including him, regardless of any personal crisis that may come up.

Smith took a deep breath, pushed back from his desk, and rose out of his chair. Just then, Ralph came around the corner.

"What happened?" he asked. "You knocked half the stuff off my shelf."

"Sorry."

"Hey, no problem," Ralph said. "This place makes me crazy, too."

"Your Energy Conservation Event will terminate in one hour," promised the voice from the ceiling. "Enjoy the natural environment."

By the time they descended the first flight of stairs, the lights went off as the main electrical service to the building was cut.

The cafeteria on the ground floor opened exactly at noon.

Most Wexler employees anticipated the power going off and arrived early. Ralph and Smith propped themselves against the wall like scolded children to wait with everyone else.

"Man, we're lucky to have Central West. I haven't heard a thing about any other work coming down the pike," Ralph commented.

"The new stimulus plan is just going into effect," Smith countered.

"Yeah, you're right. Some of that money should go to upgrading the FART system by connecting it to the subway."

"Infrastructure was number three on the President's agenda," Smith reminded his colleague.

"At least we'll be getting out of this box to do some site visits at Central West," Ralph finished.

Nodding his head in agreement, Smith thought it would be fun to be on an actual construction site for a change. In the past two years, he couldn't remember a single structure that left the drawing board for reality.

"I'll walk to the other side of town," Ralph was saying, "just to put my feet in the mud."

This comment caught Smith off-guard. For a guy who liked to complain about the smallest of things, Ralph was suddenly showing a hearty willingness to work hard. Maybe it was a ploy to find a new way to avoid actual work. After all, outside the walls of the office lurked all sorts of distractions and hiding places, all of which could be justified in clever ways.

"Here we go," Ralph said as the people ahead of them started for the door. "Let's get in there before the rest of the herd mows the field."

Smith pulled himself off the wall and followed Ralph into the cafeteria. They passed through the line where they loaded their trays with wrapped sandwiches, paper cups of macaroni salad, and tall glasses of weak iced-tea. Josh caught up with them outside, where they shared a table on the broad lawn that backed up to the building.

The last person to arrive was Lynn, the only female member of the team. Her tray featured a bowl of bran cereal, and a pocked banana. She shot Ralph a surly glare as he launched into his thick sandwich.

"What?" Ralph asked, pieces of bread tumbling out of his mouth.

"How are you going to stay under two hundred eating like that?" Lynn asked.

"I got plenty of time before the weigh-in."

Slapping a spoon into her cereal, Lynn said, "We'll see."

The spat between Lynn and Ralph never went beyond snide remarks. It centered on the quarterly Health Policy Implementation Audit. One by one, every Wexler employee received a cursory physical designed to catch the early signs of disease. After having their fingers pricked for a blood sample, Smith and his team had to step on the scale. Those persons exceeding the prescribed weight for their height paid what was called the "fat tax." Universal Coverage was funded by a flat twelve percent levy on everyone's wages. However, the fat tax cost some people between one hundred and two hundred fifty dollars more each month.

Determined to be released from this obligation, Lynn suffered through her bland lunch like a penitent nun.

Preoccupied with his unfinished report and situation with Timmy, Smith ate in silence, chewing each bite thoroughly to give himself something to do and a reason not to speak.

More than anything he wanted to hear his cell phone ring with a message from the HAO. It wasn't to be. As the other men chatted about various subjects, there came not a peep from his phone, which sat on the side of his tray.

"How's Timmy doing?" Josh asked.

"Taking it easy," Smith answered.

"Something wrong?" Lynn queried.

Hesitating, Smith told her, "He'll be fine."

No one believed their team leader. His darkened eyes, stiff countenance, and weak voice betrayed the truth.

Lynn asked, "Is it serious?"

"Very," Josh put in.

"Come on, boss. Don't keep us in the dark," Ralph said. "We're your friends."

"Let's wait for the second opinion," Smith told them. "We're all engineers, right? We know better than to rely on any single data source."

"This is your boy's health we're talking about," Lynn reminded him.

"Of course," Smith said, "I'll have the authorization for a second opinion today, and by the end of the week, I'll have a better idea of exactly what the situation is."

Lynn scoffed at this. "When did you apply for the second opinion?" she asked.

"Last week."

"You'll be lucky to have the authorization this week. Then you'll wait a lot longer before seeing a doctor."

"No," Ralph protested. "The district offices aren't that bad. A day or two more at the most. My cousin got his gall bladder notice in four days."

"Really?" Lynn countered. "When was it removed?"

Ralph shrugged. "Couple of months later."

"Probably more like six months later."

Nothing more came from Ralph.

"Let's not give the boss any more to worry about," Josh suggested. "It's not like he doesn't have enough to do already."

"It's okay," Smith said. "It'll work out for the best."

Everyone took the opportunity to sort the paper from the glass and plastic on their trays in anticipation of depositing each item into the proper recycling bin. Josh then collected these materials into neat piles on his own tray and volunteered to carry it all away.

"Thanks," Ralph said and promptly stretched out on a patch of grass beside the table. "A whole hour for lunch," he sighed. "Isn't this great?"

Smith thought that it was a pleasant diversion from the tension of the office. He remembered how he first experienced a mid-day break during a trip to Europe. It was the summer before his last year of college, interning with a multi-national firm. People working there often escaped their jobs for two hours over lunch. They relaxed at a nearby restaurant, ran errands, or met their wives, girlfriends, and sometimes both. He remembered thinking how enjoyable that lifestyle was. At present, however, he wished he could have finished his report and then made a call to the Health Admin Office. Unfortunately, he couldn't do that because, like Wexler Associates, most every business and government office except those with special licenses shut down for the simultaneous lunch hour and Energy Conservation Event. The only thing Smith could do was relax like Ralph, a master of the art. There was nothing wrong with that, Smith told himself. He was already doing all he possibly could.

Then Lynn interrupted his thoughts. "Don't wait around for that second opinion," she said. "Rose would be with me today if I had done things differently."

Rose, Lynn's sister, died of cervical cancer. It spread into her lymph glands and lungs. Nothing could be done, but Lynn blamed her death on Universal Coverage, claiming that had treatment started immediately the cancer would not have spread. It was easy to blame someone after the fact, Smith knew. Occasionally there were cases where no amount of treatment helped, no matter what the timing. He hoped this was not the case with Timmy.

"If I had to do it all over again, I'd send her to the *Salvare*," Lynn whispered.

Appalled, Smith replied, "That's an unlicensed facility. Who knows what goes on out there?"

"Like what we have is any better. Did you ask Timmy's doctor for his diploma?"

Smith was now in the position of contradicting his earlier argument with Hannah about the emergency room doctor. He was left with the choice of defending the man or admitting that he was making a mistake.

Frustrated, he said, "It could be nothing. After the second opinion, I'll know more."

"Unless it's too late," Lynn finished and got up from the table.

Too late was a term Smith understood in a completely different context. As an engineer, there was usually a work-around, a way to fix a previous mistake. Rarely was something too late to be rectified and there was always the option of demolishing what had been built and starting over. The same principals did not apply to human beings, but Smith never figured he would have to confront that reality.

Looking over the lawn, Smith wondered how many people faced similar medical problems. Everyone in sight seemed healthy and content. They chatted with each other, made jokes, a pair of guys even arm-wrestled. He couldn't be the only one. At the emergency room as well as at the Health Admin Office there had been lines, long lines. Just the same, no one here seemed to be affected, at least not enough to be talking about it.

He scanned the area until he spotted Lynn seated at a table with no one else. No doubt she was having a tough moment, mourning the loss of her sister, blaming herself (erroneously or not) for her death. Smith longed to avoid such a reality. He planned to die before his son, as he imagined every father did. Wasn't that how it was supposed to be?

He looked at his cell phone one more time and saw there were still no messages. Recognizing that there was nothing he could do at the moment, Smith put his head down and closed his eyes on an otherwise beautiful day. Given that he hadn't slept more than four hours a night for the past several days, he promptly drifted off.

Half an hour later he awoke with a start.

"Your Energy Conservation Event has ended," came the announcement. One by one, the lights in the building flickered on.

•◆• •◆• •◆•

Round the clock security had been a key selling point that made Cliffwood popular with Smith and his peers. They liked the idea of someone keeping an eye on the comings and goings of the neighborhood. However, as he entered the development, Smith managed to ignore the cluster of unruly foliage around the gatehouse. No longer attended by a uniformed person, the gate itself pointed at the sky, permanently open to anyone who wanted to pass through it. A small pile of paint chips collected around its base.

The gatehouse had been unoccupied for many years. Similarly, no one tended to the landscaping in the same period. All the common areas of the development were abandoned in the name of cost control. Residents voted to eliminate the monthly assessment to pay for such niceties. Their utility bills skyrocketed with the price of oil, as did their cost of driving to work. In any case, the neighborhood never had a crime problem, so doing away with the security guard and the landscapers was no great loss in the face of more important expenses.

Smith parked his pickup in the garage then entered the house not expecting to find anyone home. Tuesdays, Timmy stayed after school for an advanced program while Hannah worked late accordingly. Normally he treasured these quiet hours, taking the time to ruminate on whatever project he was working on or simply catch a couple hours of uninterrupted television. This evening he remained unsettled. Without the distraction of Timmy's homework or Hannah's discussion of her current candidates, he was alone with his worries. He dreaded checking his email or even the short walk to the old-fashioned mailbox.

His cell phone hadn't beeped, so Smith figured there was no message waiting for him and the odds of one in the mailbox were slim. The last piece of correspondence he received had been the registration card for his pickup. Like everything else, the fee had increased, this time from six hundred dollars to one thousand. Using a credit card, he paid it over the Internet to save the price of a stamp, which last year had been two dollars. He couldn't remember if postage was going up again or not.

He switched on the television then skipped through the channels to the all-news station. Another report about the drop in unemployment held his attention. After this bit of good news the host teased an up-coming summit of the G7 nations.

"Coordinating the stimulus plan is at the top of their agenda," the host said. "When we come back, an interview with Pennsylvania's Senator Carter, the first politician to take on the oil companies and who says an investigation is needed into the highest reaches of these mega-corporations. Senator Carter, when we come back right after this."

Two seconds of blank screen were followed by a commercial. It began with a couple clutching each other. The camera circled them, slowly moving in to show their faces, which were streaked with tears.

"Have you lost a loved one recently?" a comforting voice said. "Your loss can be the earth's gain. Consider organic burial at the Forever Green Park."

The formerly distraught couple now walked hand in hand through a meadow of wildflowers.

"Organic burial prevents dangerous chemicals from entering the biosphere. It saves valuable resources, including scarce urban real estate. Your loved one will honor the earth by fertilizing a perpetual garden that is both beautiful and environmentally beneficial. If you're considering this option for yourself, prepaid plans are available so that your family will not be saddled with an extra burden at this most painful of times. Don't forget, you may be eligible for an environmental tax credit for selecting this option."

The next commercial was for a new condominium project in South Philadelphia. "Better than the suburbs. Less crowded than center city. All the space with none of the hassle. Only blocks from the newly renovated 69th Street Subway Station. Federal housing assistance available for those who qualify."

This commercial he'd seen before. Square block after square

block of the city had been bulldozed. Two and three story row homes were replaced with four and five story multiplexes. Each floor typically housed a single family. Sometimes the top two floors were offered as a more spacious option. Like immigrants of the past, many young families choose this option. The difference was, instead of coming from another country, they were leaving the suburbs.

The third commercial forced Smith upright in his chair. The camera skimmed along the top of the ocean, then rose high into the air before looking down at a beautiful white ship. This was a luxury liner to be sure. Her hull and deck gleamed bright and clean. The glass of her balconied staterooms reflected the glowing sun. A title overlay the image:

"*Salvare*, your healthcare alternative."

Smith resisted the temptation to switch off the television, choosing to watch the message unfold, shot by shot, growing angrier with each one. Perky, fit, young women assisted patients exercising in the swimming pool. A buff young man walked beside an elderly woman whose hip had supposedly been replaced only two weeks earlier. Then came the operating theaters staffed by dozens of doctors and nurses, all busy performing life-saving tasks. A pharmacist dispensed medication into bottles for a young woman with two children. At last there was a message from Dr. Steven Jossy, Medical Director of the *Salvare*.

"Our team of obstetricians would like to welcome expectant mothers and fathers to our brand new birthing center here aboard the *Salvare*. We've taken extraordinary steps to provide the most comfortable environment, highly competent staff, and latest medical equipment to ensure the safest possible delivery of your baby. In addition, your friends and loved ones can join you as part of a package that includes twin occupancy cabins, nightly entertainment, and our chef-prepared meals."

As if the food matters so much, Smith thought. He'd like to see Dr. Jossy's credentials, which had to have come from a dubious university. As the commercial pattered along, Smith fumed at the thought of Jossy getting away with operating a private hospital aboard a ship that trolled just beyond U.S. waters. He knew that people like Jossy ruined the system for everyone. He drained the talent pool by hiring away doctors, nurses, and physical therapists, among others, who would otherwise have been employed by the Universal Coverage System. No doubt the lines would be shorter if Jossy's ship was not out there. Smith never actually inquired as to the cost of the various services *Salvare* offered, but they had to be expensive. One look at the ship and its amenities was all it took to make an accurate assumption.

What if those people worked on this side of the line? Smith wondered. How many children with conditions just like Timmy's might be better served?

"Quite a few," he said aloud.

This is what those rallies had been about, the ones Smith had been thinking of before lunch. Like his father, Smith had been on the front lines. No, he hadn't carried a gun. He hoisted a placard into the air: HEALTHCARE FOR ALL. It had been a fight and a tough one at that. Smith, Hannah, their college friends, and a good many other people believed that everyone deserved the same healthcare, no matter what their socio-economic status. Why should someone suffer, or even die, simply because they were poor? Amazingly, there were those who thought that if you didn't have the money that was your tough luck. These sentiments were never said, not aloud or in public, but they were infused into the doctrine of certain politicians, mostly those lobbied by the big insurance and pharmaceutical companies. They wanted their hefty profits regardless of who was actually served or not. These facts he gleaned from his professors and the community leaders who organized the rallies.

Thankfully, Smith's choice of candidates for president, the Senate, and the House all won that election, and subsequent ones after it. These people enacted Universal Coverage and The United States finally joined the nations of the world in securing the right to medical treatment for all its citizens.

There were always opportunists who dodged the system though. Smith despised these people, both the patients and the doctors who treated them. They thought that they were above going to a facility where everyone else went. They wanted an exclusive place, like a country club, where only people with the money to pay were permitted access. To Smith, this was nothing short of evil and the government agreed. Private medical facilities were outlawed three years ago. The *Salvare* arrived off the coast of Cape May, New Jersey, barely twelve months later.

"Come by boat or take advantage of our helicopter service, which operates nightly from the former Cape May County Airport," Jossy was saying.

"Helicopter service!" Smith groused. The cost of a single round trip was enough to pay a doctor for a month, maybe longer. "What a waste," he sighed.

The commercial ended with a glorious shot of *Salvare* cutting through placid waters as the sun set in the background. It might have been an advertisement Smith had seen for the cruise ship on which he and Hannah had spent their honeymoon. That had been a fantastic trip with stops at various Caribbean islands including St. Lucia, Martinique, Curaçao, and Aruba. More people than ever traveled by ship, but as passengers on cargo vessels, not as vacationers with nothing more than a lust for sunshine and fruity drinks. Flying was simply too expensive for most people.

"The preceding message is not endorsed by the Universal Coverage System. The medical facility mentioned is neither licensed by the United States Government, nor staffed by personnel who meet the requirements set forth in the Universal Healthcare and Medical Assistance Act, including any amendments thereto. Visiting such a facility without prior approval may result in the suspension of your Universal Coverage benefits, the assessment of a fine, and/or punishment up to but not exceeding one year in prison as determined by the Healthcare Administration Authority."

Smith almost cheered as the scene changed to the network anchor.

"Senator Lou Carter, thought of as a loose cannon by both his colleagues and the public, is best known for writing the legislation that enabled the government to take possession of the major oil companies during the last war in the Middle East. Now he contends that oil company executives continue to skim profits without paying taxes according to the same laws that govern regular American citizens. Let's join Senator Carter for his side of the story."

Having read an article about Carter's attack on the oil companies, Smith decided to forgo a live performance. He switched off the television and glanced at his cell phone. No message indicator flashed on the screen. Putting the phone away, he decided to check the mailbox, just in case there was a glitch in system.

Outside, he squinted at the empty street. Originally, he preferred quiet streets so that Timmy and his pals could play without the danger of traffic. But at present only one of Timmy's friends remained, Joe Anzalone, Jr., who was a bit of a bruiser.

The others moved away to places like the South Philly condos in the TV ad.

As he approached the mailbox, Smith refused to look farther down the sidewalk to see if any other neighbors had departed. At a cocktail party he and Hannah hosted for their fellow Cliffwood residents, everyone in attendance swore they wouldn't move back to the city no matter how expensive gas became. And then several families did just that, disappearing in the middle of the afternoon without taking the time to say goodbye let alone leave a forwarding address. Truth be told, Smith frequently considered whether it was better to follow them out or hold on.

Opening the mailbox he was stunned to see a letter inside. It was from Health Administration District Office 117. He tore it open, slid out a sheet of paper, and read the contents. To be sure he hadn't made a mistake he read the letter a second time.

"This is bullshit!" he hollered and stomped up the driveway.

Timmy passed through the kitchen, walked directly to his room, and slammed the door shut. He didn't want to talk to anyone, least of all his parents. His pals at school called him everything from a sissy to mommy's boy because he no longer rode the bus with them. He was "special" because he couldn't play at recess and was exempt from gym class. They made rhymes about him that had the girls in stitches. To make things worse, when he told his mom what happened she said that she was going to talk to the principal to put a stop to this bullying immediately. Was she crazy? If she spoke to the principal, Timmy knew he'd be doomed.

"You're overreacting," his mother insisted. "After a little talk with the principal everything will be fine."

"No!"

"Keep your voice down," she said. "You have a serious condition, Timmy, and it's not right that other kids treat you badly because of it."

"Just let me ride the bus, mom," he pleaded.

"Out of the question," she replied. "If something happens at school, the nurse is there. You don't have that luxury on the bus."

"Nothing's going to happen. I feel fine. Without some batting practice I'll never make the starting team this summer."

"Put your head back and take ten deep breaths in a row before you say another word."

"But ..."

"Timmy, I mean it."

It was no use. Frustrated, he bounced his head off the seat a couple of times.

"That's enough," his mother said, deepening her voice. "You're going to aggravate your condition. Is that what you want to do?"

"I want to ride the bus!" he hollered.

His mother refused to talk to him for the remainder of the journey home. No sooner had she switched off the vehicle than he hopped out of the car and bolted for his room. He knew better than to ask for help from his dad, who always agreed with his mother when it came to things like this.

Smith heard Timmy's door bang. "What's going on?" he shouted.

Just then Hannah entered from the hallway into his study. "Is there anyone in this house who can speak in a normal tone of voice?" she asked. She took in the expanse of her husband's desk, which was covered with file folders, pages from a book that had been cut to pieces, and several colored markers.

"We have a big problem," Smith began.

"You're right. The kids at school are humiliating Timmy because he's not riding the bus anymore."

"Humiliating?" Smith questioned.

"That's right," Hannah said. "I'm going to speak with the principal tomorrow morning and put a stop to it. This kind of bullying is terrible for his self image."

"It'll pass."

"We're in an uncaring mood this evening," she remarked.

"Actually, I'm doing my best to get Timmy a second opinion somewhere closer than Mars."

Hannah spun on her heel and exited the room.

"Where are you going?" Smith called after her. Rising out of his chair, he caught the edge of his desk, tilted it forward, and spilled some of the paper onto the floor. "Damn it," he said and left the mess for later.

He caught up with his wife in the kitchen where she stood before the open refrigerator.

"I'm not speaking to anyone in this house unless they're going to be polite," Hannah greeted him.

"Okay," Smith said after a breath. "The second opinion authorization came today."

Smiling sweetly, she said, "That's wonderful."

He handed her the letter, remarking, "Not quite."

An appointment for Timothy Smith has been scheduled with Dr. H.Z. Khawaja on June 22nd at 10:15 AM.

Hannah looked up and said, "I don't see the problem."

"Please, read a little further," Smith urged.

The Pittsburgh Health Administration District Center for Pediatric Medicine is located at the corner of 3rd Avenue and Wood Street.

It took a few seconds for Hannah to absorb this next piece of information. Her eyes continued down the page, taking in the rest of the contents as if there had been nothing amiss in the previous paragraph.

If you are unable to keep the assigned appointment, please notify this office immediately. Appointments canceled one week or more before the appointment will not cause a penalty. Any appointment canceled within one week or less without approval is subject to a fine of two hundred fifty dollars. The same applies to missed appointments which are not validated. The local Health Administration District Office reserves the right to alter the schedule according to circumstances that may arise on or before the day of your visit. Please come prepared with all appropriate documentation, including proper identification and your Universal Coverage Card.

Just then it occurred to Hannah that if Timmy was going to see Dr. H.Z. Khawaja, he would have to travel to Pittsburgh.

"There has to be a mistake," she said evenly. "Give them a call tomorrow, explain that we live in Philadelphia, and I'm sure they'll find a doctor right here."

"You can bet I'll be doing that," Smith assured her. "In the meantime ..."

"Your voice is turning hard, Bob," Hannah put in.

Mellowing his tone, Smith began again. "I've been examining the Universal Coverage Manual. I'm working out exactly what our rights are."

"You mean Timmy's rights," she corrected.

"Exactly. Timmy's rights. He's the patient, but he's just a boy. It's up to us to see that things are done properly. I'll be damned if ..."

"You're starting to sound like your father."

He didn't appreciate the jibe. His father may have used some foul language from time to time but he'd been a good father, a veteran, and a respected small businessman. He was nothing like those oil executives Senator Carter was going after or, heaven forbid, Dr. Jossy, who might have been a snake oil salesman in a previous life.

"I'll be at the Health Admin Office tomorrow morning, bright and early. I'm not going to let anyone put my son at the back of the line."

"Absolutely not," Hannah agreed.

"I CAN'T ANSWER THAT QUESTION WITHOUT MORE DATA."

CHAPTER SIX

ROBERT SMITH THOUGHT OF HIMSELF as a highly educated individual, a hard-working member of the upper-middle class, and a generally good person. He'd never been the type to cut corners or abuse the system, whichever one it happened to be. Didn't he forgo his sick days when he could have used them for vacation? Didn't he strictly adhere to the carpooling regulations? Didn't he wait his turn at the fuel depot without a complaint? He was even careful around the coffee pot at work, making sure he didn't contribute to the mess.

Nonetheless, he recognized when he had to get his hands dirty. As his father told him, "Sometimes you have to reach into a bucket of oil to get the tool you dropped." In this mode, he left a message with Wexler Associates' Human Resources Department that he was too ill to go to work today. Then he called Josh to say the same thing, and when pressed for details, related only that the problem was intestinal.

Smith loaded his pickup with everything he needed for a successful trip to the Health Admin Office: cash to bribe the guard, a folding chair to wait in line, and his indexed, collated, and highlighted pages of the Universal Coverage Manual should there be any question about healthcare policy.

He was excited enough about his prospects to skip breakfast, settling for nothing but a cup of coffee. Before leaving the house, he told his son it was only a matter of time before he would be back on the bus.

"Promise, dad?" Timmy asked.

"I promise," Smith replied, adding that smart boys ignored bullies, listened to what their teachers said, and treated their mothers with respect.

Having decided to play the game for what it was, Smith thought he could win. He might make some mistakes along the way but he was armed with the Universal Coverage Manual, not to mention plain old common sense and reasonableness. As he drove to the HAO, he couldn't help but believe that someone made a mistake in assigning Timmy a doctor in Pittsburgh, something as simple as a pair of numbers reversed in the zip code. For this reason, he kept his attitude positive and reminded himself about Hannah's insistence he not overreact.

"Timmy takes in everything you say and do," she said as he went out the door. "If you act like a blowhard, he'll act like one, too."

She actually used the word "blowhard." When did he ever behave that way? In line with her instructions, he kept his cool, kissing her on the cheek to show that he was paying attention.

As he parked his pickup, he noted that he made record time even though he coasted as much as possible. He went so far as to switch off the engine as soon as he entered the parking lot, allowing the truck to roll along in neutral until the front tires bumped the block bordering an empty space. He expected another medical emergency gasoline voucher, but wasn't above saving fuel in any way he could. Not only did it help the family budget, it also protected the environment. Despite a few things on this particular day, Smith did the right thing to the best of his abilities. Like Hannah said, he was setting an example for Timmy the way his father had set an example for him. He wanted his son to be part of the world's solutions, not part of the problems.

Approaching the front door, Smith spotted the guard on the other side of the glass. He wasn't exactly sure how to offer the man and his boss some money for special consideration or how much was required. He continued forward, wiping his hands on his pants, before pulling open the door and stepping inside.

"This facility is closed," the guard sneered. "What do you want?"

Smith almost turned on his heel and walked back outside. Then a flash of anger took hold, one that nearly prompted him to start explaining to this guard that he was acting like the kids who bullied Timmy. Instead, he redirected his indignation by reading the nametag on his adversary's uniform.

"Officer Plant," Smith began, "how are you this morning?" Had his voice squeaked? He hoped not.

"Tired," Plant replied. "Been up all night staring at these walls."

"Sorry to hear that. I'd like to talk to you about the line."

"Rieser runs the day shift. He's the one who deals with the line."

Feeling brave, Smith asked, "Are you sure about that?"

Plant squinted at Smith as he said, "Well, if someone were to find a note under a block outside it might get passed on to Rieser. You follow me?"

Although he nodded his head, Smith was not sure that he understood.

"You going to stand there all day or get out of the way so I can do my job?"

"Sorry," Smith said, backing toward the door.

Outside, he moved along the sidewalk wondering what he should do. Then he remembered how last week Plant had come out of the building and poked around the weeds for a few seconds. Sure enough, just a few feet away, Smith discovered a concrete block. The question was how much money to leave? Five dollars? No, that paid for a can of Coca-Cola, a candy bar, and not much else. Twenty dollars? That seemed like a lot, but how much was his time worth? At last he lifted the block a few inches and peeked underneath. There he saw several notes with fifty-dollar bills attached lying in the dirt.

Smith replaced the block and trotted to his pickup. There he wrote B. SMITH on a scrap of paper, clipped it to five ten-dollar bills, and folded the combination into a tight rectangle. After a quick glance toward the door, he retraced his steps to the concrete block where he deposited his contribution to Rieser.

Fifty dollars was more than twice the co-pay he'd made in the days before Universal Coverage went into full effect. On the other hand, he hadn't paid anything for Timmy to visit the emergency room or for the ambulance ride, and nor would he open his wallet for the inevitable second opinion and whatever treatment followed. All this and more was covered by the twelve percent Healthcare Premium assessed on every citizen's income. He couldn't imagine what the *Salvare* would charge for such amenities. It had to be in the tens of thousands. Therefore, fifty dollars for a spot near the front of the line seemed like a bargain.

As the line formed, Smith took his place, leaving his chair on the back of the pickup. He figured he wouldn't need it and he wasn't disappointed. Plant and Rieser came through as advertised, assigning him the sixth spot. Smith felt a tinge of shame as he weaved among the less fortunate who had to wait their turn. He wondered if it was because they were ignorant of the guards' scheme or lacked the funds. Either way, he vowed to report these malefactors to the powers that be, which was the best he could do for the others and a bit of penance for himself, too. First, he had to deal with Timmy's condition. He entered the office fully prepared to do just that.

With three specialists on duty, Smith waited only twenty minutes before taking a seat across the desk from Ms. Olga Buckley. She yawned without covering her mouth, took a few seconds to examine her cell phone, and finally focused on her client.

"How can I help you today?" she said at last.

"I'm here to reschedule my son's appointment for a second opinion," Smith told her.

"Reschedule?" Buckley queried. Her diffident manner left no doubt about her opinion of such a request.

Anticipating such a reaction, Smith grinned with satisfaction that he had not only memorized his petition but rehearsed it as well. He said in a tone that would have met Hannah's approval, "According to Section 109 of the Universal Coverage Manual, *a client is permitted immediate application for rescheduling in the case of extreme risk, undue hardship, or as I believe has happened, in the event of an error on the part of a Health Administration Service Professional.*"

"Are you saying I screwed up?" Buckley retorted.

"Not you specifically," Smith answered diplomatically, tilting his head over a slight shrug. He reveled in her attack. It meant that he had won the opening round of what might be a longer bout. "No," he continued with the same gentle tone, "I'm sure there was a simple clerical data entry ..."

"Stop right there," Buckley interrupted him. "Not only are you saying I screwed up, you're referring to me as some kind of clerk, like an old lady making change at a convenience store."

"No," Smith said raising his hand like a crossing guard.

"I'm a Healthcare Administration Professional, grade H 14. You know what it takes to get a job behind this desk?"

"Please ..."

"Please listen to me, mister whatever your name is. Don't march in here thinking you're going to talk that way to someone in my position. Is that clear?"

Having dealt with a few client outbursts at Wexler Associates, Smith knew better than to respond verbally. Instead he nodded his head with neither a smile nor a frown. He assumed a neutral posture in the chair, folding his hands over his stack of files. If he was going to salvage the meeting, he needed to steer back onto Timmy's case or he would lose any chance of getting what he wanted.

"My son Timmy has been diagnosed with a defective heart valve," Smith said quietly.

"Not the first one I've heard about in this district," Buckley said.

"Then you know how serious this condition can be."

"Doesn't give you the right to barge in here looking for special treatment."

No it doesn't, Smith almost said. He checked that answer

UNIVERSAL COVERAGE 101

and took a moment to evaluate just where he stood. This woman appeared to enjoy arguing with him, watching him play the grateful, soft-spoken, needy client while she lorded her authority over him. To continue on this tack would get him nothing. Therefore, he played the strongest card in his hand, the one he hoped would be a last resort.

"Ms. Buckley," he said, "I'm working on a CGP, a Critical Government Project. I'm not at work today, missing very important meetings during which my input is absolutely necessary. I would be there, guiding this project along its proper course if it wasn't for the dire condition of my son. Any father in this situation would miss a day at work no questions asked. So, I'm not saying there's anything special about me or my son, aside of a tiny error made by someone regarding my son's second opinion and further treatment. If you'll help me straighten that out, I'll be out of here and back to work where I belong."

The conviction with which he told this half-lie impressed Ms. Buckley and Smith himself. Not wanting to leave any doubt that he would do whatever it took to clear up this mess, Smith revealed to his host just how well-acquainted he was with the Universal Coverage Manual.

"Under Section 508, Ms. Buckley, Critical Government Project employees take precedence over those whose cases which fall under the regular rules found in Section 102. I'm not invoking my rights under Section 508 even though I could if I wanted to. I just want to correct this little error and get back to my team at work. I'm sure you understand."

"Let me call my supervisor," Buckley said. "It's better if she handles a 508 directly."

"Thank you."

Ms. Buckley's supervisor stood barely five foot tall, wore a jacket over her shoulders, and hung a pair of glasses on a chain around her neck. Her name was Ellen Ledsoe and Smith estimated her age close to his own, somewhere in the mid-30's. She managed a smile and waved for Smith to follow her down the hall to a corner office twice the size of the one he surrendered to help Wexler Associates meet their energy conservation goal.

Inside, he found the temperature cold enough to store ice cream, which explained the jacket over Ms. Ledsoe's shoulders. Smith took a moment to close the door so as not to share his problems with anyone passing by. Then he sat down opposite Ledsoe who busied herself with her own chair, which seemed to be stuck in a position too low for her satisfaction. She pressed on a lever while pulling on the base until it was fully extended. After a quick grin she took her place and rolled forward only to find her knees level with her desktop.

"Tell me what brings you to me, Mr. Smith," Ledsoe said.

"A second opinion has been scheduled for my son," Smith explained. "The problem is, the doctor is in Pittsburgh."

"Let me see your documents," Ledsoe said next.

Smith placed the second opinion authorization on the desk then leaned back.

Ledsoe lifted her glasses to the edge of her nose then glared over them at her visitor. "I mean all your documents, Mr. Smith," she said. "Start with your Universal Coverage Card and don't stop until the last piece of paper that came before this authorization."

From his wallet Smith took his UC card then produced the paperwork from Timmy's visit to the hospital as well as the copy of the form he filled out to request the second opinion authorization. He arranged them neatly on Ledsoe's desk in chronological order.

Ledsoe first examined his UC card. "This is out of date," she said. "Where's your new one?"

"On the way," Smith replied, making a mental note to request a new one as soon as he got home. It struck him as odd that a card was required when everyone was entitled to care. Why have one?

"Hmm ..." Ledsoe muttered, "Heart valve defect. This district has had quite a few of those lately. My own theory is that some congenital defects are related to long-term exposure to the exhaust from internal combustion engines. One more problem the previous generation dropped on us."

Hearing that Ledsoe had been working on a theory, Smith said, "I didn't know you were a doctor."

She let her glasses drop. "I'm an Administrative Systems Analyst, Mr. Smith, a graduate of the Kennedy School of Government and attendee of countless seminars at Harvard's Center for Federal Efficiency. I don't allow myself to be limited by the knowledge of the medical profession, which as anyone who sees what I see every day knows is trapped in the past."

Smith wondered if there was anything he could say to this lady, or anyone in the building for that matter, that wouldn't provoke a hostile reaction. He thought it best to stay focused and paid Ledsoe a compliment to move things along.

"I feel fortunate to have you helping me with my son's situation."

"My job is to analyze requests for medical services and to be sure the resources that provide those services are allocated in the most efficient manner. I'm not permitted to 'help' anyone with a particular problem. That would be unfair to all the others. Analyze and allocate, those are my prescribed tasks. I take them very seriously."

Nodding in total agreement, Smith felt like his first impressions of this woman were off the mark. His knowledge of engineering naturally included efficiency. As for fairness, he was a consummate practitioner of the concept in his position of team leader. Like him, she had a job to do, and that she was focused on doing it seriously and properly comforted him.

He waited patiently while Ledsoe reviewed Timmy's paperwork, glancing at the framed certificates on the wall, many of which confirmed that she had indeed attended many seminars. She also received commendations for not missing a single day of work in half a decade. Plus, she was a volunteer at a number of groups from homeless shelters to an organization called Mothers Without Fathers.

Smith and Hannah drifted away from their causes after moving to the suburbs, especially after Timmy came along. Yet they did their part, responding to a call the President and Congress made through the American Volunteer Initiative Act, which required all college students receiving federal financial aid to be registered with the National Community Outreach Bureau and to serve on an NCOB project for at least one hundred hours per year. Elementary, Middle, and High School students were also drafted into the effort and given a monthly quota of hours to be devoted to a sub-program called America Serves America. It was a great concept, one that gave Timmy an opportunity to learn the importance of volunteering at a young age. The best part about ASA was that it also offered adult citizens the opportunity to go beyond the required service in exchange for fuel vouchers, tax breaks, and even paid vacation days.

"Alright, Mr. Smith," Ledsoe said, twisting away from her computer screen. "I've examined all the particulars of your son's case. The good news is that you are employed on a CGP. That opens up the slot with Dr. Khawaja, one you might not have gotten for at least four months assuming the current system demand. The bad news is there are no openings any closer than Pittsburgh until October."

"October," Smith repeated quietly. Timmy would be in the midst of another school year by then.

"That's correct."

"But under Section 508 ..."

Ledsoe smiled and promptly interrupted Smith's plea. "Yes, you are employed on a Critical Government Project. I verified that through your Social Security Number with the Bureau of Infrastructure and Industry."

Smith sat up straight, perturbed at her not taking his word on the subject. Did she think he was a liar or like one of the fraudsters who cut the line downstairs?

"However," Ledsoe was saying, "the CGP on which you are employed is a state-level project."

"That's right," Smith put in. "Central West."

"Then it will be easy for you to understand, Mr. Smith, that Section 508 has both a federal and state sub-section. Included within the state sub-section is the provision to grant you one of the priority slots allocated to state-level CGP employees."

At this point, Smith wanted to take out his notes and review what she was telling him. While it sounded perfectly logical and may in fact be accurate, he didn't remember the sub-sections of 508. Upon seeing that CGP employees were entitled to priority appointments, he stopped reading, having applied his yellow highlighter to the sentence that spelled this out. He regretted not going deeper into the text.

"Are you with me so far?" Ledsoe asked.

"Yes," Smith replied.

"Good. Well, then we're finished. Your son has an appointment with Dr. Khawaja next week, which I must say is quite soon given the caseload the system currently faces."

It took a few seconds for Smith to absorb what he'd been told. Then the engineer in him kicked in and offered an alternative. "What about in New Jersey or Delaware or even New York City or Washington, D.C.? Aren't there any openings there or someplace in between?"

"In the first place, no one is permitted to enter the New York or Washington Health Administration Districts for care without a Federal approval. As for New Jersey and Delaware, they are regions separate from this one, which is part of the Pennsylvania Directorate. You would have to apply for an appointment at an HAO within those districts. As you are not a resident of those districts, the System Specialists there may summarily deny your request."

"Is it more efficient for me to drive 350 miles to Pittsburgh to see a doctor instead of maybe 35 or less to New Jersey or Delaware?" Smith inquired.

With amazing confidence, Ledsoe answered, "Without a doubt it is," adding with a look over her glasses, "in the context of the system."

For all the disappointment that Smith felt settling in his gut, he had to admit Ledsoe was correct. Of course this didn't mean he was willing to accept the verdict, at least not without a fight. The question was how to wage that battle without losing the war. He forced himself to consider that Timmy's health was more important than anything, including his ego.

"I find it hard to believe there are no appointments closer to Philadelphia," he said at last.

"There are appointments," Ledsoe countered, "You simply have to be patient. Ms. Buckley could easily assign your son one at a renowned Philadelphia hospital. As I said, there are a few slots in the October timeframe, but the system worked perfectly by overriding that and granting you a position much sooner, albeit in Pittsburgh."

Those two sentences crystallized his situation. He could wait four months, hoping Timmy would be okay the whole time. Or, he could go through the expense of driving to Pittsburgh only to discover that the emergency room doctor had correctly diagnosed the problem. Then what? As long as he had a Health Administration Specialist in front of him, he decided to ask.

"What happens after the second opinion?" Smith queried.

"I can't answer that question without more data," Ledsoe answered.

"More data?"

"After a second opinion confirms or contradicts the first opinion, a course of treatment may or may not be prescribed. If treatment is prescribed, it will have to be provided by the system, the demands on which we won't know until the time of the request. It varies from day to day, sometimes from moment to moment."

Smith shifted in his seat and pressed on. "Let's say the second opinion confirms that my son needs a heart valve replacement. What happens then?"

"As I have already explained, the request will be handled at the time it is presented and scheduled accordingly," Ledsoe said.

"And if that request came today?"

Growing impatient, she said, "I am not permitted to speculate on the location, timing, or expected outcome of any care-related issue," and began gathering together Smith's papers on her desk.

He was about to give up when an idea occurred to him. "What if someone in the area cancels?" he asked.

"No one cancels," came the reply, "unless Code 4CE applies,

in which case every name on the waiting list moves up."

"Code 4CE?"

"The death of a client."

Although his question had been innocent, Smith blanched at her answer. He noticed that Ledsoe had just put his UC card atop the stack of papers on her desk and gently pushed them to his side.

Before accepting her dismissal, Smith inquired of a few more details. He began with, "Is there any assistance available to pay travel expenses related to medical emergencies?"

"There is, but your case does not feature an emergency code, nor does your income level permit you to benefit from that program."

"How do you know?" he blurted before he realized what he was saying.

"Section 1214 of the UC Manual. *The Health Administration Office shall have access to the tax records of all clients and their authorized and/or certified caregivers in order to equalize service opportunities among clients with varying incomes.*"

"You automatically access these records?"

"Not me, the computer. I only analyze the data." To make the point, she tapped her index finger atop the stack of paper that waited for him atop her desk.

Presented with his documents in a neat bundle, Smith found himself with no more questions. He took his papers, slipped them into his folio, and smiled for his host. Knowing that he might face her across this desk again, he wanted to leave her with a positive impression.

"Thank you," he said genially.

"My pleasure," Ledsoe replied, wiping her hand across a now-empty desk.

CHAPTER
SEVEN

IT WASN'T UNTIL HE WAS THREE-QUARTERS of the way home that Smith came to terms with what a waste his morning had been. Not only had he failed to secure a closer and sooner appointment for Timmy, he missed an important day at work and burned several gallons of gasoline. What was he supposed to do for the rest of the day? He couldn't show up at the office, not after calling out sick. He wasn't about to go for a ride because Ledsoe did not grant him a gasoline voucher. Still, he had to try everything within the system to do the best for Timmy, and that meant a long, expensive trip to Pittsburgh.

He scolded himself for being a selfish, petulant, ingrate at the HAO. Overtly, he came across as a nice guy, aside of that business about Section 508. He'd been a bit arrogant about his position on a CGP and as a team leader. Luckily, Hannah had not been there, or he would have suffered another reprimand. Pulling into Cliffwood, he pondered whether she might be correct in her analysis of latent thoughts he picked up from his father, who had certainly been a confident, and at times, demanding person.

Smith reminded himself that the HAO people had jobs to do and they were doing them well. After all, his CGP status had been figured into the equation automatically, which is why Timmy's appointment was scheduled for next week instead of four months. He should have been pleased and humbled by the privilege that his son had this opportunity when so many others might not. Similarly, there could be a good reason for sending him to Pittsburgh. Perhaps the medical center there specialized in heart ailments. He should have asked more questions about the facility instead of angling on how to get to the front of the line. In a way, his approach had been as devious as those bribing Rieser.

The question of transporting Timmy to Pittsburgh remained. Getting to the other side of Pennsylvania would take time and money. This wasn't like during the First Iraq War when Smith and some college buddies traveled to Carnegie Mellon University for an engineering competition. They piled into an old sedan and drove straight across the state, 350 miles on the Pennsylvania Turnpike, paying the nearly thirty dollar toll mostly in quarters, dimes, and nickels as a joke. He didn't know what the current fee was, probably four times that. And the gas, back then it had been three fifteen a gallon, a price everyone complained about. Compared to today it had been a bargain.

Thankfully, the President was talking about intercity rail as a new priority, just like healthcare had been. Rebuilding a system that had been all but dismantled during the previous forty years would take time. No matter, it would come. If anyone could make it happen, this President could. In the process, Wexler Associates would no doubt design portions of the required infrastructure. Therefore, Smith had two reasons to thank this President: for his job and for the thousands of dollars it would surely cost to fix Timmy's heart.

Feeling better about the whole situation, Smith turned into his driveway only to find a moving truck parked down the block. His first friend in the development, the man who swore he would be the last to leave and then only in a coffin, Joe Anzalone, Sr., carried a dining room chair to the side of the truck. Hopping out of the pickup, Smith rushed down the sidewalk, and confronted his neighbor's betrayal.

"The last to leave, eh?" Smith said, catching Anzalone on his way back to the house.

"It wasn't my decision," Anzalone countered.

"Really? Who decided for you?"

"Keep it down, would you?"

"Who's going to hear us?" Smith said, bristling.

Anzalone stopped in his tracks, turned sideways to Smith, and said, "Let's go across the street and hash this out?"

"Sure," Smith agreed. It occurred to him that in the last several days he'd never felt so much anger. First at the emergency room, then at work, next at the HAO, and now with a guy he'd known for ten years. All through high school and college he hadn't been in a single fight and here he was clenching his fists, red-faced, and thinking horrible things as if he belonged to a street gang.

"I had no desire to leave Cliffwood whatsoever," Anzalone

explained. "I still don't, but Jenna heard about a great deal near 64th and Lindbergh, a two-floor, three-bath, with a balcony. It comes with a zero percent incentive mortgage and the Federal Green Initiative Stipend, which pays my moving expenses if I agree to junk one of our cars."

"When did that get started?" Smith asked.

"I don't know. You got to be looking all the time, which Jenna was. She surfs the builders' websites, calls the banks, checks in with the Government. All of them. This is her thing, Bob. She's been wanting to get out of here ever since Brenda and Harry moved out two years ago. When Tina and Sam hit the road, she fell into a depression that had me scared. Forget about Little Joe, he's having problems because there's no kids around here."

"There's Timmy. He and Joey are friends. They play on the same team."

"Yeah, and I feel sorry about leaving like this, but what am I supposed to do? You want me to put up with my wife in tears every night? My kid throwing rocks through windows to work out his frustration? What would you do?"

"I'd wait until school was over," Smith put in.

"Soon the schools here are going to lose all their special programs," continued Anzalone. "Then they'll cut the sports. There might not be a baseball team next year. In the city, they have a stadium for the kids at Little Joe's new school that looks like something the Phillies should be playing in. He's there meeting the coach right now."

Once again, the argument made too much sense for Smith not to admit he was wrong. Anzalone was doing the right thing for his family, even if he was abandoning his friends and the neighborhood.

"You still promised me you'd stick around," he said weakly.

"I did, and I'm sorry, Bob. Believe me, I feel like a schmuck skating away in the middle of the day when everyone else is working. You have to cut me a break on this one, though, because I have no choice."

"I understand," Smith heard himself say. Anzalone patted him on the back and shook his hand. Embarrassed by his own diatribe, Smith recalled how awkward he'd felt around the President.

"Look, the Green Initiative only pays for four hours with this truck, and I get twenty-five bucks cash for every fifteen minutes less. I'll call you when we get settled in. You and Hannah can come over for dinner or something. Bring Timmy. Little Joe would like that."

"I will," Smith replied reflexively as Anzalone moved toward Cliffwood's next soon to be vacant house.

Peeved at his friend's broken promise, Smith retreated to the garage. At least Anzalone hadn't asked him to help load the truck, which would have been an unforgiveable insult. The man had that much class, even if he was playing the coward by sneaking away without informing his neighbors.

Although the day continued to be a disappointment, Smith wasn't about to let Anzalone's departure get under his skin. He set about organizing his garage, a task he'd been putting off for months, one that would earn him points with Hannah. First, he installed a set of hooks high on the wall. On these he placed Timmy's new bike, knowing that it may take a while, but sooner or later his son would ride it without worrying about anything other than traffic. As light as traffic was these days, that was a small concern.

Next came the multitude of little things that gathered over time. There were two five-gallon plastic jugs for gasoline. He used these for his lawnmower before the gas-powered type had been outlawed. He put them in the middle of the floor, vowing to fill them even though hoarding gasoline was illegal. Now more than ever, he wanted to store some fuel in case of another emergency with Timmy. He was willing to risk the fine; the police weren't likely to check his garage. Then he pulled his toolboxes out of the far corner and placed them next to the gas jugs. These were actually his father's toolboxes.

"Never give up your tools," his father had said. Smith kept them, understanding that they were handy, expensive, and a memorial to his father.

Next, he cleared the narrow workbench of some miscellaneous items, hung a pair of pliers on the adjacent pegboard, and discarded some old newspapers in the recycling bin. What had he been saving those for? It was a question he wouldn't hear from Hannah again now that they were in the trash.

He was ready to sweep the floor when he took a second look at the newspapers. There on the front page was the reason he kept them. "22nd AMENDMENT REPEALED. PRESIDENT TO RUN FOR THIRD TERM." Spreading the pages over his workbench, Smith read the article carefully. He remembered the day when this newspaper landed in the driveway. Both he and Hannah celebrated with champagne because this man had been the only president of their adulthood. He was the longest serving president since Franklin Delano Roosevelt, who presided over equally challenging times.

Smith flushed with pride at having changed the nation. It would be wrong to throw this newspaper away, especially now that the news came only via the Internet. Printed copies no longer existed and entire forests had been saved. It was an irreplaceable piece of history, a sacred document that needed to be preserved for when Timmy was an adult.

He found a pair of scissors, neatly cut the article from the rest of the paper, and placed it on the side of the workbench. Only after he finished did he check the other side of the page. He saw that he'd clipped through another headline, one equally dramatic. "UNIVERSAL COVERAGE TO ABSORB PRIVATE INSURERS." In smaller text below was, "HOSPITALS, DOC PRACTICES, LABS TO FOLLOW NEXT YEAR." Another article bore the pull quote, "PHARMACEUTICAL COMPANIES VOW FIGHT."

Smith nodded his head. He had been part of history, even if it was only one vote. Two if he counted Hannah's. Both of them, like so many other Americans, finally listened to reason, and made sure that everyone had access to high-quality healthcare without going bankrupt. Fortunately, this had taken place before Timmy's problem appeared. Otherwise, what would they have done? He might have discovered his private policy had obscure exceptions, conditions that were partially covered, or those that weren't covered at all. He could have ended up broke like that woman in the TV commercial during the election. He might be in the street not because he was moving to the city like Joe Anzalone but because the bank foreclosed on his house after he spent the mortgage payments on doctors and hospitals. Was he better off with a slight delay or with the chance of losing it all?

Luckily, he didn't have to answer that question. He busied himself finishing his chores until the garage was ready for his Chief Master Sergeant father's inspection. His dad would have been proud, too. There was a place for everything and everything was in its place. Finally, he carried his newspaper clippings into his home office where he dropped them into a brand new folder where they would rest until it was time to explain to Timmy how bad things used to be.

Coming out of his office, Smith decided not to tell Hannah anything about Anzalone moving or Timmy's appointment. He wanted to have a nice family supper, an opportunity to bond with his family, the people he loved more than anyone else. There was nothing he could do about the Anzalones or Timmy's next appointment, so why not make the best of it?

Make the best of it he did. No sooner had Hannah and Timmy come through the door than Smith took his son back outside for a chat. He spoke with the cool manner of a baseball team's manager making a visit to the pitcher's mound. The first topic was those kids at school, whom Timmy should ignore because he had door-to-door service like a big league player and they had to ride the bus like a bunch of guys on the farm team. Next came the news of the Anzalone family's departure.

Upon hearing that Joey was gone, Timmy refused to cry. He had an ache in his chest, a hundred times worse than the ones that came and went once in a while. But a champion didn't cry, not even when he committed an error that cost the game. He went back to the dugout, took his lumps, and practiced hard until the next game. The problem was that Joe Anzalone, Jr., his teammate and friend, would not be at practice, not that Timmy himself was allowed to take the field either.

"We need Joey on the Moguls this summer," Timmy pleaded. "He's our best outfielder."

"I know," Smith said, "but look at it this way, another kid will get a chance to fill the spot."

Was his dad kidding? The other kids weren't as good as Joey. They were too slow or couldn't keep their eye on the ball. How could they win with a hole in the outfield?

"He should've told me," Timmy said.

"Don't blame Joey. His mom and dad probably didn't tell him until the last minute."

"Why wouldn't they tell him?"

"Sometimes people have to make difficult choices," Smith answered, embarrassed by his lack of honesty. "I'm sure he'll give you a call soon."

"Yeah," drawled Timmy, who knew his team couldn't win with two of its best players off the field.

We have to get out of here, Smith thought. If he found a place close to the Anzalones, Timmy and Joey would be back on the same team, playing in that beautiful stadium.

"Let me show you where I put your bike," he said to distract his son from the bad news.

"I can't reach it," Timmy said, looking up at the place of honor where his bike now hung in the garage.

"You're growing faster than you realize," Smith replied. "By the time you're tall enough to get it yourself, I'll be teaching you to drive."

The gleam in his son's eyes gave Smith more satisfaction than landing his position as foundation team leader at Wexler Associates. No doubt the doctor in Pittsburgh would properly diagnose Timmy's problem and that determination would have him on the road to a permanent recovery. How long could the delays be? Not long enough to affect his son's long-term future.

Returning to the house, Smith implored his son not to share their conversation with his mother. The news about the Anzalones Smith wanted to reveal himself, when the time was right.

"This is between us."

"Okay, dad."

For the rest of the night, Smith wanted to relax on the couch, watch *On The Prowl* with Timmy, and not worry about things that were beyond his control. With some minor effort he was able to achieve his goal.

Hannah picked up on his attitude. She went so far as to ask if he'd gotten a raise or something, but Smith brushed her questions aside with platitudes about how good they had it compared to all the less fortunate.

He and Timmy took up their stations on opposite ends of the couch, Smith with coffee, Timmy with a glass of juice. Right on time, *On The Prowl* began, this episode featuring a story about a thief who stole a very valuable baseball card from a museum. Just as a critical clue was discovered the screen went blank.

"AWWWWW!" Timmy whined. "No fair."

The Seal of the President of the United States came on then dissolved away to a view of the nation's chief executive seated in the Oval Office. A man of the people, the President sat cross-legged and in his shirtsleeves on the end of a couch instead of stiffly behind his desk. Smith appreciated the gesture, feeling that the man was without the pretensions of his predecessors. He was the embodiment of equality, a regular guy instead of a pretender. After all, who wore a jacket while sitting on his couch at this hour?

"I bring good news to the nation this evening," began the President.

"Not now," Timmy complained. "I want to see how Elroy caught that sneaky thief."

"Shhhh!" Smith said. "The President is speaking. Remember what I told you about respecting people of authority?"

"The Federal Energy Management Board has reviewed this month's statistics and has determined that gasoline stocks are sufficiently high to allow an increase in next month's ration allotments as well as a decrease in the price per gallon. I feel this demonstrates conclusively that federal energy management policy is working effectively and to the benefit of everyone. However, my administration will continue to push Congress for more investment in mass transit. Our cities have never been better served than they are today, but there is always more work to be done. I need your support, your continued commitment, to making this happen."

Better news could not have come to Bob Smith on this particular night. Getting Timmy to Pittsburgh would be a little cheaper and those mass transit projects were the kind of jobs Wexler Associates could handle.

After a pause, the President said, "I won't keep you any longer. The networks have been very gracious in holding their shows so we won't miss a single moment. Good night, America, and rest assured your government is working for you. Don't forget, if each of us sacrifices a little, everyone will have more."

"Did you hear that?" Smith called over his shoulder to Hannah.

"What?"

"Just another reason to be happy," Smith replied.

◆— • •◆— • •◆— •

During the drive to work, Smith couldn't have been more upbeat. He and Josh reveled in the President's news. Sure, the gas ration only amounted to another two gallons per month. Nonetheless, it was two gallons more as opposed to two gallons less the way it had been over the winter. And the price had dropped.

"I'm going to put a few gallons aside," Josh said. "Maybe

Mindy and I will head to the mountains this summer."

Smith thought about the empty five gallon jugs he had in his own garage and wondered how many people had similar ones in defiance of the anti-hoarding law. There were probably mayonnaise jars and olive oil tins filled with the stuff in every neighborhood, which made for a dangerous fire hazard. Luckily his house was a fair distance from the others.

Switching gears, Smith busied himself calculating how much gas he would need to get to Pittsburgh and back. The round trip was approximately seven hundred miles. Assuming twenty-eight miles per gallon in Hannah's vehicle, he needed twenty-five gallons. That was the minimum. It was also more than half his month's ration, actually closer to two thirds. How was he going to save that many coupons by next week? It was impossible. He would have to apply to the local Motor Fuel Management Bureau to receive an advance on his allotment for a hardship case, which would be easy with all of Timmy's paperwork. Thankfully, the HAO letters bore official stamps and signatures that would be more convincing than simply filling out a form.

"Don't miss the turn," Josh said, snapping Smith out of his reverie. "You okay?"

"I'm fine," Smith answered. He cursed himself for not thinking the problem all the way through yesterday. He could have gone to the fuel depot for a fuel advance application instead of cleaning the garage.

"Good morning," Ralph said to Smith when he arrived at the coffee station. "Tell me you wouldn't like to have some behind-the-dugout seats for the Phillies versus the Mets."

"You have to win a lottery to get those," Smith commented.

"Yeah, unless you're a friend of a friend. You know what I mean?"

Under an arched eyebrow, Smith said, "You'd have to be friends with the mayor to get those seats."

"Or someone I know," Ralph said, waving two tickets in his free hand.

Amazed, Smith inquired how he managed to get the tickets, and more importantly, how could he afford them.

"You got to know people who can do you a favor at a reasonable price."

"A reasonable price?" Smith asked. "How much is that?"

"Depends on what you're looking for. Everyone gets a little piece, but hey, nothing's for nothing, right?"

Two guys from another floor poured coffee and simultaneously listened to Ralph prattle on about his skills as a purveyor of hard to obtain items.

"You ever want to take Hannah to a concert, just let me know," he said to Smith. "It'll cost you a small premium, but I deliver nothing but the best."

"I'll keep that in mind," Smith told his co-worker. "How about getting on the phone and finding out when those test boring results are going to be in."

After a look at his watch, Ralph replied, "Two minutes, boss, then my time is your time."

Smith arrived at his cube to find the message light flashing on his phone. It was from Henny Geerman who asked that he come to see her as soon as possible. Since he needed the test results before he could do any more work, Smith decided to visit Geerman immediately so as not to interrupt his flow later in the day.

Geerman anxiously arranged things on her desk as Smith

settled into a chair. He couldn't imagine her getting this bothered over his vacation days.

"I received a message from your HAO late yesterday. It was an official notice, Bob."

Before Smith could react to this statement, Geerman continued, wringing her hands as she spoke.

"It's a 56E, a Confirmation of a Life-Threatening Condition. I had no idea what you were facing."

Catching up, Smith said, "It might not be. He's going for a second opinion next week."

"That's encouraging. Be aware, this has to be dealt with correctly, and I have to admit Lynn Kessler's case was the only other one like it."

"Lynn never told me she had a problem," Smith said.

"Not Lynn, her sister, Rose. Lynn isn't married and has no children, so the Universal Coverage System requires her employer to administrate the healthcare of her next of kin who are unemployed, which prevents the other agencies from being overloaded. Just thinking about what happened to Rose has me upset about Timmy."

Smith found himself in the strange position of comforting Geerman when perhaps it should have been the other way around. Regardless, he appreciated her empathy and informed her that Timmy was doing well, taking it easy the way he was supposed to.

"I want you to know that I'm going to do everything I can to be sure this is handled properly."

"Thanks, Mrs. Geerman," Smith said brightly, thinking that maybe she could find a way to get him a few extra gasoline vouchers.

"I have to check through the guidelines and regulations for you," she said. "I'm going to make sure you get every benefit you're entitled to."

"That sounds great."

"It's the least I can do, Bob. It may take Mr. Wexler's approval but you're getting the max."

CHAPTER
EIGHT

IN SHORT ORDER, Ralph secured the test boring results for Central West. They only confirmed that Smith's earlier analysis had been correct: a conventional foundation would be inadequate to support the residential towers. This meant that a more sophisticated system of interlocking cells of steel sheets filled with concrete would have to be built. Smith had done this previously for a chemical company and the nearby oil refineries. He reveled in being right for a change, especially in light of his bouts with Hannah and the Health Admin Office.

As the daily Energy Conservation Event began, Smith and his team were already on their way down the stairs. They took to their usual table, eating and chatting about the visits they would soon be making to Central West. The conversation ran out with the food. Each person emptied their tray and took a position away from his fellows. Ralph stretched out for his nap, Josh mixed in with a group of secretaries, and Lynn wandered off to an empty spot of lawn for her daily prayer.

Team Leader Bob Smith remained alone at the table, pondering how he was going to tell his wife about taking Timmy to Pittsburgh. He wished he could ask a favor of Doctor Ben. Maybe he could call a friend or a colleague who might wrangle an appointment closer to home, but that was just another form of cutting the line. If everyone did it, the system disintegrated into chaos. He reminded himself to solve the whole problem, the next piece of which was obtaining the gasoline for the trip.

Given his workload, the hours rushed by. Smith finalized a preliminary report about the Central West foundations, one he intended to give to Mark Wexler. He compressed the details into a few pages, which was no easy feat. He carried this to the pickup at the end of the day, handing it to Josh before turning the key.

"Read over this tonight and we'll discuss it in the morning. If everything looks good, we'll hand it to Mr. Wexler tomorrow afternoon."

Having thumbed to the conclusions section, Josh whistled through his teeth. "He's not going to like this," he reflected.

"We can't change the results of the last ice age," Smith returned. "If he wants twenty-five storey buildings, he doesn't have a choice."

"He did say twenty-five."

Smith turned out of the parking lot saying, "Double-check it. Make sure it's right."

"I will," Josh agreed then added, "Is Timmy going to play in the summer league?"

Catching himself before he automatically gave the wrong answer, Smith said, "Maybe he can keep the stats."

"That's a good idea. It will keep him involved with the team."

It wasn't as important as being the best hitter and the fastest base runner, but it was a job that had to be done. Smith nodded his head reflexively, switched on the classical station, and continued in silence. He made a brief stop at the fuel depot to grab two copies of the Application for Fuel Ration Advance.

Fifteen minutes later he pulled to a halt in front of Josh's house at Briarwood.

"See you tomorrow," Josh said slipping out of his seat.

Just as the passenger door closed, Smith noticed his preliminary report on the console between the seats. "Hey!" he called to his co-worker. "You forgot something."

"Oh, yeah," Josh replied with a grin and caught the report Smith tossed to him.

The Fuel Ration Advance paperwork occupied Smith for half an hour. Filling in the boxes, he realized that his commute was going to be less convenient. His regular gas allotment would be spent taking Timmy to Pittsburgh, so he'd have to park his pickup and endure the FART for ten additional round trips. If Anzalone hadn't moved away, he might have caught a ride with him and then taken the subway to the Wexler building. Smith shook his head, muttering about his former neighbor's betrayal. It was selfishly ugly of the man to bail out without fair warning.

Before Smith could dwell on this injustice, Timmy and Hannah arrived, both of them in reasonably good spirits that carried all the way through supper. Smith himself managed to keep his mood upbeat even as he fretted over telling Hannah about Pittsburgh.

"Am I going to play for the Moguls this year, dad?" Timmy asked.

"You'll be there," Smith answered even as he scrambled for a way to tell his son that he wouldn't be able to play the game. Who knows, if the doctor in Pittsburgh contradicted the one in the emergency room, Timmy might be able to take his place among the other kids and possibly score the winning run the way Smith imagined he would.

Taking the opportunity to break the news about Pittsburgh in a positive way, Smith said, "After a check up in Pittsburgh, you'll be on the field hitting one grand slam after another."

"Pittsburgh?" Timmy repeated.

"There are some good doctors there, son. One of them is going to make sure you're ready to play this summer. You don't want to let your team down, do you?"

"No."

"Of course not. Most kids are lucky to get to the Poconos for a week of camp. You're getting a trip all the way to Pittsburgh."

"Are we taking the pickup?" Timmy wanted to know.

"Your mother's SUV gets better mileage."

"You're going with us, right?"

"I have a big project at work."

"So do I," Hannah muttered. "Your father and I have to discuss this, Timmy."

His mother's tone was not lost on Timmy. A discussion meant that he was either in trouble or that he had to do something he didn't want to.

"I'm finished," he said even though several bites remained on his plate.

Sensing his son's anguish, Smith said, "Let me get your bike."

Timmy leapt out of his seat and bolted for the garage.

"Why didn't you tell me about Pittsburgh?" Hannah asked from behind a wicked glare.

"I just heard from the HAO today," he lied.

"What about the gas?"

"I'm dropping off the application for an advance at the fuel depot tomorrow. Have you heard back about the M Fuel Supplement Card we're supposed to get as part of the UC benefits?"

"Not yet," Hannah replied.

"Dad!" Timmy called from the garage. "Let's go!"

"We're going to talk about this trip to Pittsburgh later tonight," Hannah warned.

"Thanks to my position on a CGP we have the appointment in Pittsburgh, honey. If we don't take it, Timmy will have to wait until October."

Shaking her head, Hannah said, "I still think we're overreacting. Timmy seems fine. He probably just exhausted himself. All this panic will do nothing but ruin his self esteem."

"Come on, dad!"

As Smith walked along the pavement, Timmy literally rode gentle circles around him. His son's strength and ability revealed no trace of an underlying ailment. Standing on the pedals, Timmy whipped in close, then leveled out and coasted for several dozen yards before repeating the process again and again. The boy didn't so much as break a sweat. Smith could not help but think that Hannah might be correct; maybe they were overreacting.

"Go easy, Timmy," Smith warned his son. As an engineer, he knew it was always better to err on the side of caution rather than to push things to the limit. He wallowed in the comfort of knowing that the second opinion would be issued by a specialist as opposed to a harried emergency room jack of all trades.

A swath of trees, probably part of the original forest from which Cliffwood had been carved, stood at the end of the development. This hundred-yard-deep "green space" separated Smith and his neighbors from the homes of Briarwood, where Josh lived. A trail cut through the woods, one kids from both sides used to travel to visit each other. With Little Joe gone, Timmy was alone as Smith did not want him traipsing through the forest by himself.

"Let's head home," Smith told Timmy.

"Okay, dad," Timmy replied, slipping off the seat. He guided his bike by the handlebars, keeping pace with his father's easy gait.

No sooner had Smith hung the bicycle on its newly installed hooks than he heard a vehicle pulling into the driveway behind him. Both he and Timmy turned to see a shining Chevrolet grille facing them.

Doctor Ben exited his pickup with a broad smile. He crossed the driveway in a few bounds and said, "You're easy to find in this ghost town."

"How's that?" Smith asked.

"Just look for the first house with signs of life," Ben joked, adding with a hand extended toward Timmy, "I'm Doctor Ben."

"My name's Timmy."

"Pleased to meet you, Timmy," Ben replied.

"What brings you all the way over here?" Smith asked next.

Ben placed his bag on the workbench then explained he was visiting a patient at the edge of his district and thought he might as well stop by to see how Timmy was doing.

"I appreciate that," Smith said.

"The least I can do," Ben put in.

Timmy watched as Doctor Ben opened his bag, took out a

stethoscope, and draped it around his neck. Despite the man's imposing figure, he wasn't the least bit afraid. Unlike the emergency room doctor, who kept sighing and grunting, Ben spoke clearly and directly. His eyes were steady and bright, not the least bit shifty the way that fellow at the hospital had been. Thus, when asked to hop onto the workbench so Ben could listen to his heart, Timmy readily complied.

"I'm not a cardiologist, but I know a good ticker when I hear one," Doctor Ben said as he stood beside Timmy ready to place his stethoscope to the boy's chest.

Everyone's attention swung to the side door as Hannah's voice suddenly filled the garage. "What's going on in here?" she demanded.

"Doctor Ben stopped by to listen to Timmy's heart," Smith said somewhat more casually than he intended.

"Doctor Ben?" Hannah questioned. "Doctor Ben who?"

"He was a customer at my father's station. He's also a Designated Visiting Physician for District 128."

"A visiting physician, too?" Hannah scoffed.

Taken aback, Smith flushed with embarrassment. Just as he opened his mouth to allay Hannah's skepticism, she cut him off.

"Timmy," she said, "go to your room." When Timmy hesitated, she stepped between her son and Doctor Ben, taking the boy's arm and tugging him off the bench.

"Listen, honey, Doctor Ben is doing us a favor," Smith said, not forgetting to use his calm voice.

After a deep breath and quick glance to be sure Timmy was in the house, Hannah said directly to Doctor Ben, "Excuse me, but I don't know you."

"If it will help, let me show you my license," Ben offered,

"Those fat cats have been draining off the profits while guys like us get nothing. Gas would probably be a dollar or two cheaper if it wasn't for their big salaries."

"More like three or four dollars less a gallon," the clerk said.

"Whatever. Who says they should make a couple million bucks a year when some people can hardly afford to pay for twenty gallons a month?"

"Right on," the clerk affirmed

"Senator Carter and the President. What a team! They know how to put people in their place," his boss said. "They got those doctors in line, and we're not talking about at the Mercedes dealership either."

"The drug companies, too. No more pills that cost fifty bucks a pop. We all get them for nothing now."

Smith appreciated their sentiment, but he was anxious to get to work. "I'll stop by on my way home," he interjected. "Sound good?"

"No problem, Mr. uh … Smith," the administrator replied after a glance at the first line of the application. "We'll have your vouchers here in an official envelope. And, hey, good luck with the trip to Pittsburgh. I hope your boy turns out to be just fine."

Mark Wexler called a meeting of everyone involved with Central West. They piled into the company's largest conference room that resembled a movie theatre. Smith sat with his team in the back row, an appropriate spot for the foundation department.

"This morning, the governor called me personally," Wexler began.

A worried buzz rose from the attendees. Was their company president about to announce the project had been canceled and consequently that many of them were going to be laid off? Impossible. The President had just given it his seal of approval. Then again, some of the older attendees had been through that drill before.

His hands up for the crowd to be quiet, Wexler said, "The governor is going to make a visit to Central West for the ceremonial first shovel."

The room erupted with a cheer. Their jobs were safe.

"There's plenty of work to be done, especially by you members of the foundation department seated in the back."

All eyes turned on Smith and his team.

"The governor wants hard numbers to pass on to Pennsylvania's congressional delegation. Everyone here is counting on you guys to hit the mark the first time. The governor told me he's not going to get a second chance on the funding. We get what we get from this session's stimulus bill. After that, we're on our own."

Smith shifted in his seat. He was confident he could have a thorough analysis and a subsequently detailed report finished by the end of next week. He'd already begun the process. Still, all those eyes on him were nerve wracking.

"There's more good news," Wexler was saying. The governor revealed some of the details from his monthly meeting with the President. He said in not so many words that what we here in this room all know: that this President has been pushing for mass transit since he took office three elections ago. No surprise there, right? Well, he has two years to go and he wants a legacy in rails and stations."

"You mean he's not running for a fourth term?" someone called out.

After a heavy wink, Wexler said, "I'll pass that question up the ladder. What the governor wanted me to know is that there's going to be requests for proposals in the intercity transit sector like never before. The most important ones are going to be fast-tracked by the President and his friends in Congress so the shovels hit the ground about a year from now."

"Just in time for the campaign to begin," a voice shouted.

Someone else said, "If he connects the FART to the subway, I'll start a petition to make him president for life."

"Settle down," Wexler told the group. "We're here to provide engineering solutions to whoever happens to be in office. Let's stay focused on that and not get distracted by politics."

Back in his cube Smith began dividing the work among his team. He considered each person's strengths and did his best to assign the tasks accordingly. It wasn't long before Ralph showed up.

"Can we step into the stairwell for a private meeting?" he asked.

"Maybe at the end of the day," Smith suggested.

"This is important," Ralph said. "It's about Central West."

In the stairwell, after checking to be sure no one was above or below them, Ralph informed Smith that he was taking some unplanned vacation time the following week.

"I can't allow that," Smith said firmly, "not with the governor coming to town."

"Listen, boss, I'm doing you a favor by giving you notice. What if I just called out sick the way you did the other day?"

"That was a real emergency, Ralph."

"Like you would have known the difference if I made the call next week and didn't show up."

"I can't believe you'd do this when you know what's at stake."

Ralph stood his ground. "Give me some credit," he said. "You want me to work over the weekend, I will. You want me to stay late the rest of this week, I'll do that, too. But I got a week coming in Ocean City, a place on the beach, the whole deal. There's a new woman in the mix. That's the hardest part to rearrange, and she may be able to help you."

"Wait a minute," Smith said, moving closer and lowering his voice. "How did you get the gas to drive all the way to Ocean City and back?" Josh held a more senior position and he was struggling to accumulate the fuel to make a similar trip.

Backing up a little, Ralph answered, "I have my sources."

"I'll say. Can't you reschedule in a couple weeks?"

"She's not going to wait," Ralph said. "You must have missed the part about how she can help you. She works for the Health-care Administration Authority, on one of the oversight commit-tees. Give me time to get to know her and she can juggle the schedule for whatever Timmy might need. You follow me?"

He did but despised himself for considering the type of deal Ralph was proposing.

"I'd never cut out on you," Ralph pleaded. "Give me what you need to get done and it'll be on your desk in record time. Let me make it worth your while?"

"Are you trying to bribe me?"

"It's not a bribe; it's a consideration. Besides, I'm not shirking my duty, I'm simply rearranging when it's going to be done. How many other guys in this building can deliver the work on time and a little bonus for those who understand flexibility? Eh? And if there is somebody else like me, I'll bet they don't have a chick with pull in the right places like the one I'll be dancing with."

Smith couldn't believe he was hearing this argument. He should have fired Ralph on the spot, or at least put a written reprimand in his permanent file.

"A ten-gallon gas voucher at the Essington Fuel Depot Ralph said, barely whispering, "which just so happens to be on your way in and out of the city."

Ten gallons would guarantee Smith enough fuel to take Timmy on another journey for treatment. Therefore, he accepted Ralph's bid with the caveat that all his assigned work had to be done by Sunday night.

"You drive a hard bargain," Ralph said with a grin and stuck out his hand.

It turned out to be an honest one at that. Ralph went so far as to bring a battery back-up device from home. He smuggled it up the stairs, plugged in his computer, and worked through the lunchtime Energy Conservation Event. When the power went off at the end of the day and everyone filed out of the building, Ralph remained behind. No one saw him at the coffee station the next morning either.

"Who built a fire under him?" Lynn asked, referring to Ralph's newfound work ethic.

The others at the lunch table shook their heads. Used to Ralph taking his mid-day nap on the grass, they were amazed their colleague had skipped what had been his favorite part of the day.

By Friday morning, Smith was reviewing high-quality work he didn't expect to see until the following week. If Ralph had behaved this way before, he might have had the number two spot on the team instead of Josh. Smith reminded himself that Ralph only performed at this level because there was something special in it for him. If not for Timmy's condition, the matter might have gone the other way. But there was nothing he could do about the circumstances, which Ralph seemed happy to exploit for his own benefit. In any case, his assigned tasks were completed early, and it would only make Smith look better in the eyes of Mr. Wexler that his team performed under pressure.

Toward the end of the day there was one thing left for the team that week: their quarterly health maintenance checkup. They met at the entrance to the cafeteria, where Ralph was first in line. He bounced on his toes, threw imaginary punches, and sucked air like he was drowning.

"It's not going to help," Lynn warned.

"Speak for yourself, my lady."

"I'm two pounds under, mister."

"On whose scale?"

"The one that matters."

"We're about to find out," Ralph said as he was waved in with the rest of the bunch.

The visiting nurse was a lanky fellow who wore a white smock over sweatpants. His nametag identified him as Reggie. With him was a Care Delivery Specialist who handled the official paperwork. She introduced herself as Megan.

Reading from a card, Megan explained the process. They'd all heard it before but it was her job to repeat it so no one could claim their rights had been violated or that they had been treated unfairly.

"The quarterly health maintenance checkup is provided free of charge," Megan began. "The goal is to catch early signs of disease, such as …"

"Yeah, yeah, we heard all this before," Lynn interjected. "Let's get it over with."

"She's right," Ralph seconded. "I'll go first."

"I have to read the entire paragraph or I'll be in violation of Section 2233, Part E."

"Tell you what," Lynn said, "I'll say that we all heard it from the horse's mouth, and he'll swear to it." Her finger pointed at Ralph.

"Scout's honor," Ralph offered.

"But ..."

"Take the chair," Reggie said, unwrapping the blood pressure cuff. Megan retreated to a chair next to him.

Ralph sat down next to the nurse, rolling up his sleeve on the way. As the cuff inflated he slowly closed his eyes.

"One twenty-six over seventy. Normal," announced Reggie.

"He's anything but that," Lynn remarked.

"Please, no comments," Megan piped up. "You can be reprimanded for hurtful speech."

After Reggie pricked Ralph's finger for a blood sugar test, he stepped onto the scale. Ralph glanced over his shoulder and stuck out his tongue at Lynn. She rolled her eyes as Reggie read the numbers.

"One ninety ... seven ... eight ... nine ... two hundred ... no, one ninety eight and a half."

Megan entered the weight into a space on the form.

"No freaking way," Lynn grumbled as she sat down for the blood pressure cuff. She passed that but not by as wide a margin as Ralph. Then came the finger stick, which made her yelp. At last, she tiptoed onto the scale.

"One hundred forty one ... two ... wait ... one hundred forty one and a quarter."

"Made it!" shouted Lynn.

"By a mere twelve ounces," Ralph called back.

"Doesn't matter. You're buying the first round."

Thanks to Ralph's assay of the test boring data, Smith had everything he needed to make good use of the weekend preparing his foundation plan revisions. Across his desk at home, he spread a diagram of the Central West site. Contour lines defined the extent and shading denoted the depth of the various soil layers. Using a sheet of tracing paper, he overlaid the footprint of the three towers, making sure it was properly aligned with the existing streets.

"What are you working on dad?" Timmy said from the doorway.

"Something strong to hold these buildings," Smith answered.

"Yeah? Like what?"

Smith explained to Timmy how difficult it was to build something on top of mud. To create a stable platform on which the buildings would stand, a series of steel legs had to be pressed down into the ground.

"How do you do that?" Timmy wanted to know.

"With a pile driver. It's like a giant hammer that pounds a long sheet of steel into the soil. Each sheet of steel interlocks with the next one. You place them in a big circle until the first one connects to the last one. When it's finished it's called a cell, just like a cell in your body. Then you dig out the mud and fill it with concrete."

"Wow. That sounds heavy," Timmy commented.

"It's heavy," Smith agreed, "and strong, too. After you have a bunch of cells built, you can put a skyscraper on top of them."

"Let's give your father some peace and quiet," Hannah suggested as she put her hand on Timmy's shoulder.

The weekend evaporated as Smith refined his ideas. He had the house to himself after Hannah accompanied Timmy to his monthly America Serves America outing to ensure he wouldn't do anything strenuous. They traveled to a northwest corner of Philadelphia where they gathered trash from vacant lots on Saturday. On Sunday, they joined a group of high-school students fulfilling their own service requirement by painting the exteriors

"I'm going to drop in on some friends in the city," Josh said. "They can give me a ride home. Worse comes to worst, I'll take the FART."

"You sure?"

Josh put out an open hand. "Let me save you a few steps," he said. "I'll deliver the report and you can head out."

His keys were in his pocket and there was nothing else at his desk that he needed, so Smith waved to Josh and turned for the parking lot. In the lower lobby, he came across Lynn again.

"Hear anything about Timmy?" she asked.

Smith looked at his watch, saw that it was still an hour before Timmy's scheduled appointment, and shook his head. "Maybe in an hour or two."

"Don't fool around," Lynn returned. "No matter what the second opinion is, I'd have him on the *Salvare* as soon as possible."

It perplexed Smith why an otherwise intelligent woman fell for promises made by a slick huckster like Dr. Jossy. In the years since the *Salvare* arrived off the coast of New Jersey, Smith heard a few rumors about people who received treatment aboard the ship, but nothing solid. He reckoned only those with big incomes could afford to avail themselves of that option. The people Smith encountered were on roughly the same income level as he was and probably couldn't afford the amenities Jossy advertised. He took umbrage at how the rich managed to get around whatever system was put in place for the greater good.

Smith took his keys out of his pocket. As much as he wanted to tell Lynn that she should get over her loss and move on with life, he couldn't do it. He never wanted to hear the same words if something horrible happened to Timmy.

"You need a ride?" he asked.

"I'm going to walk," she replied. "Maybe the exercise will burn off that Coke I drank at lunch."

The Essington Fuel Depot catered more to trucks than passenger vehicles. This made sense given its location just off Interstate 95. A convoy of tractor-trailers filled the holding pen. Each truck's fuel tank held in excess of a hundred gallons, some as much as two hundred gallons, making them likely targets for highway bandits. Hence they traveled in packs, sometimes with police escorts paid for by the trucking companies.

Smith found no one in line for gasoline and presented the ten-gallon voucher Ralph had given him to the clerk behind the glass, whose nametag identified him as Dwight.

"Ten gallons of gasoline," Dwight said, looking over the voucher. "Going on a trip or something?"

Already nervous about using an illegally obtained voucher, Smith struggled to answer. "My … uh … son has to go for medical treatment."

"Oh, yeah? You have to check out the M Fuel Supplement Card. It's a federal program connected to the Universal Coverage System, an extra fuel ration at a discounted price for people with health problems."

"My wife just got it," Smith replied.

"Good. My sister has one, too. She's a little kooky. Has to go to the shrink three times a week or she freaks out. She gets another eight gallons a month, maybe twelve, I'm not sure. Point is that it's better she burns the gas than goes off the deep end. Eh?"

"I hope she gets better," Smith said politely.

Dwight rolled his eyes. "She's nuts. Flat out bonkers. I'm stuck with her as long as she doesn't do anything dangerous."

He pounded the form with his stamp, slipped a chit in the coding machine, and entered the appropriate information into his computer. A few seconds later, he slid Smith's receipt and coded chit through the slot, taking one hundred four dollars in exchange.

"Have a good day," Dwight said and waved with Smith's money still in his hand.

Leaving the depot, Smith saw several heavily armed men guarding the trucks that had recently been fueled. They looked more like soldiers than policemen. Each one carried a submachine gun, sported a harness with spare magazines of bullets, and wore a helmet. He pressed on the pedal a little harder than normal to get away from the scene. The last thing he wanted was to get caught in the crossfire between these guys and a band of criminals.

"Bob Smith calling."

Doctor Ben's voice boomed over the cell. "Tell me you're on your way," he said.

"I am," Smith confirmed, holding the phone a few inches from his ear. "If you're free."

"You're too late for lunch but come out anyway. I'm still on the Thorpe Estate. Remember where that is?"

"I do."

Smith looked forward to the visit even though he would have to make an uncomfortable apology and most likely turn down Ben's job offer. Something about the man appealed to Smith. It might have been his defiance of the guard at the fuel depot or the kindness he showed by stopping in to have a look at Timmy. Beyond that, he literally exuded energy the way some of his college professors had. Smith was used to the dull expressions of too many of his colleagues. Lynn was forever depressed and grumpy. Josh was frequently daydreaming. Ralph seemed to be the most animated but only because he sought a sneaky way to get something for himself.

To a degree, he couldn't blame them. The economy had been in the doldrums for nearly a decade, resulting in drastic changes to everyone's lifestyle. Adjusting required time and patience, both of which occasionally ran short. Hadn't he lost his cool with Joe Anzalone? He had, and over what? Because his neighbor was doing his best to adapt to the circumstances. His judgment had been hasty and erroneous, two things any good engineer must always avoid.

At any rate, Smith was excited to spend an hour with a high-spirited person.

Turning between the stone pillars marking the entrance to the Thorpe Estate, Smith vowed to visit the Anzalones in their new apartment. While there he intended to make polite inquiries regarding the availability of similar apartments. It might be time to cut his losses the way Joe had and get out of the suburbs. It would be fun to take Timmy to Central West while it was under construction and it would be much easier via the subway than having to drive and park. Cheaper, too.

As he rolled to a stop before a handsome stone colonial farmhouse, Smith considered that he might just take whatever work Doctor Ben had for him. The extra money would go a long way to fund the plan that was slowly forming in his head. With summer approaching, it was the perfect time for Timmy to change schools. If he could find a place near the Anzalone's, Timmy would not be a stranger in his new school; Little Joe would be there to show him around. The boys could be teammates again, playing in that beautiful stadium. He knew Hannah would support the move as it would cut her commute to probably fifteen minutes and put her that much closer to her friends and co-workers, not to mention the social scene she preferred. Finally, Smith wondered if he might find better doctors in Philadelphia's Health Administration District. If so, the decision was all but made.

Four dormers projected from the roof of Doctor Ben's house. The slate roof itself stretched over the two-story structure, which featured a door in the center and symmetrical windows on each level. The mortar between the stones had been recently pointed and the paint on the wood trim gleamed fresh in the afternoon sun. Aside of its three-hundred-year-old style, the house appeared to have been finished yesterday.

No one answered the door when Smith knocked. He walked around the house in the direction of a barn and some outbuildings. He noted green cornstalks growing in the surrounding fields. During his childhood he frequently passed the Thorpe Estate but didn't remember ever seeing any crops grown. Approaching the barn he saw a fenced garden that occupied about half an acre. Doctor Ben was just closing the gate.

"Hello there!" Smith called out. Doctor Ben acknowledged his presence with a wave, and moments later the two men shook hands.

"Welcome to my humble domain," Doctor Ben said.

Taking in the expanse of fields, buildings, and care with which it was all tended, Smith replied, "A beautiful place."

"Thank you, Bob. Let's walk out back where I'll show you what I want to complete before the summer ends."

"Lead the way."

They passed along the edge of a field, the steepness of the grade slowly increasing. A dirt road marked the boundary be-

tween the corn and a patch of forest that occupied a sort of pla-
teau. Doctor Ben led his visitor into the woods along a path bor-
dered by stout oak, maple, and walnut trees, none smaller than
two feet in diameter.

Smith breathed hard as he struggled to keep up with his
host. He scanned left and right, searching for an opening among
the foliage that would give him an idea of how large this patch
of forest was. However, he found himself falling behind and
gave up his analysis in order to keep pace with Doctor Ben, who
showed no signs of his age when it came to tramping through the
woods.

At last they broke out of the trees, stopping at the edge of a
hollow that descended into a wrinkle of the landscape.

"There she is," Doctor Ben said, gesturing with his cane.

Following his host's pointer, Smith discerned the remains
of a gristmill tucked into the fold of the hollow. The roof had
fallen in and the stream that fed it tumbled through a dilapidated sluice.

Sensing Smith's assessment, Doctor Ben said, "She needs
some work, but I have a good crew coming. Before we go down
there, let me show you the feed pond."

They skirted the hollow and rambled up over a gentle hill
before exiting the trees surrounding what seemed more like a
swamp than a pond.

"I'm going to dredge that out," Ben explained, "then enlarge
it out to the west. It needs to be at least twice as big, maybe bigger, and as deep as is practical."

"You have your work cut out for you," commented Smith.

"So do you."

"Me?"

"Who else?" Doctor Ben prodded and again set off at his

brisk pace.

They took another path. This one followed the stream, led down through the hollow, and ended at the sluice that fed the mill's waterwheel. From this vantage point, Smith saw the rotted wheel had collapsed, its pieces sticking up like dinosaur bones. Built of the same stone as the farmhouse, the mill itself appeared in sorry condition. Not even a door hung at the entrance and a few stones had dislodged from the walls. The place was the perfect setting for a romantic painting, offering all the charm of a fallen castle.

"The rains are coming in fall," Doctor Ben said. "I want this thing operating by then."

"You better hire the right contractor," Smith advised.

"I have the right people. What I don't have is a bona fide engineer like yourself who can put his slide rule to use and figure out exactly how these things fit together."

"You're looking for someone to make sure the contractor does a good job, like a supervising engineer?" Smith asked.

"I'm not worried about them. I want to get the most out of the pond up there. I want to rebuild the mill and have it spinning, Bob, as much as possible."

"To process grain?"

"Among other things," Doctor Ben answered.

The trouble was that Smith was a civil, not a mechanical engineer, and the latter was what Ben truly needed.

"I can get you the names of several people who would be interested in helping you here," he said.

"Are you saying you can't handle the job?" Ben asked.

"Well, I'm a civil engineer not a mechanical one."

"Good enough. This old mill must be sitting on a foundation of some kind and the guts of it have to be fastened down properly."

"It's not that simple."

"Not that simple?" Doctor Ben scoffed. "I'll bet you this mill ran for a hundred years tended by people who might not have been lucky enough to attend the sixth grade."

Smith caught himself smirking at Doctor Ben's veracity.

"Nothing I said was funny."

"I'm sorry. You're right. There are people who specialize in historical work. They're the ones you want to talk to."

"You've described the perfect scenario," Doctor Ben said. "But do you know what that requires?"

"Quite a bit of money," Smith replied.

"The money is the least of it."

"You'll need permits, too."

On this reply Doctor Ben turned his back and left Smith wondering what he'd said to offend his host.

Doctor Ben wiped his shoes before entering the house. Smith did the same and followed him into the kitchen where a basket of apples sat in the middle of the table. From a cabinet drawer Ben retrieved a knife then settled onto a chair and began slicing one.

"Here's how I look it, Bob. Rain falls from the sky, gathers in that pond up there, and flows downhill the way nature demands it must. That I stick a wheel in the middle of it has nothing to do with anyone other than me and the raindrops. The government sees it differently. They want to tell me how to channel the water, what kind of wheel I can have, what all of it is supposed to look like according to some committee or other. For the grace of this approval, I must pay fees so that I can have a piece of paper hanging on the wall granting me permission to use the rain that falls out of the sky."

Shaking his head at the ridiculous nature of the argument, Smith said, "Don't be silly. You know as well as I that we can't have people damming up streams and rivers wherever they please."

"Unless the government says so," Ben noted, "just like they tell you where to get your gas and your doctor."

"That's not the point …"

"They sent your son to Pittsburgh, didn't they?"

With this fact, Smith could not argue.

"Did you ever ask yourself why?"

"I know why," Smith said bravely. "Care demands have to be balanced with available resources."

Doctor Ben stared at him for a long moment then said, "And that makes perfect sense to you, doesn't it?"

Unsure of what he'd missed, Smith instantly felt stupid and annoyed. He intended to give Doctor Ben a courtesy call, thank him for stopping by, and maybe offer an apology for Hannah's brusque behavior. While Smith found him amiable enough, he showed a gruff side that was more than a little unpleasant. Smith saw it at the fuel depot and now here at his home. He attributed it to the man's age and generation, both of which were as behind the times as printed newspapers. The best thing he could do was make a graceful exit and leave Doctor Ben to his fate.

"I should be going," Smith said, rising off his chair.

"Think about my offer."

"You didn't make an offer."

"I'm paying cash to skilled people," Ben clarified. "It will be worth your while."

"Thanks, but no thanks," Smith replied. "Good luck."

The man sat back in his chair. Smith thought he saw a smirk on the executive's face. He considered that thousands of doctors could be hired for three billion dollars and more than a few heart clinics could be built, too. Timmy would have been in the care of a Philadelphia doctor if these guys weren't skimming the money off the top.

"Three billion dollars represents the shareholders return on their investment," Senator Carter continued. "I want to take this opportunity to remind each and every one of you on that side of the table that this government is the largest shareholder in your company. Fifty-one percent of that three billion dollars belongs to the people of the United States of America."

From this fact Smith deduced the explanation for the President's announced reduction in the gasoline price and an increase in the monthly ration. If things continued, he would be re-elected in another landslide. Who could compete with cheaper gas and more jobs? Satisfied that things were going the right way, Smith continued through the channels until he came to a travel show extolling the virtues of Philadelphia's historic sites. Growing up in the area, he knew them well and couldn't wait to take Timmy to visit them.

The next commercial began with a view of a ship he'd seen before. Smith reached for his cell phone to try Hannah again. Before hearing the first ring, the commercial's narrator drew his attention.

"No waiting lines aboard *Salvare*," Dr. Jossy promised. "No Care Delivery Specialists between you and the physician of your choice."

"Give me a break," Smith muttered. This very day, his son had seen a doctor and had waited not two weeks for the privilege. If his condition had been worse, Timmy would have been rushed to a Philadelphia heart specialist in a matter of hours. As it was, the system had done well for him without any extra expense or worry about how to find the right doctor. The people at the HAO might not be the most cordial but they were good at their jobs, seeing to it that patients connected with the appropriate providers of care.

"Why not relax aboard a beautiful ship after our doctors provide you the most advanced treatment for your ..."

Smith wiped Jossy off the screen with a tap of the remote. He'd had enough of that guy. He reminded him of the oil company executive facing off with Senator Carter. Both wore a con man's smile, the kind that belied an inside joke. Smith hoped Carter would take on Jossy when he finished with those oil tycoons. He felt like sending an email to suggest just that. Carter frequently mentioned the notes he received from constituents.

Smith ditched the idea and swung his feet over the arm of the couch. He managed to doze off and didn't wake up until his cell phone chirped. Snatching it off the end table he saw that he had missed a call.

"Good news. Timmy is going to be fine. I'll explain everything in the morning. We're on our way home. Don't wait up," Hannah's recorded voice said.

"Take that, Dr. Jossy!" Smith cheered.

He warmed a can of soup, read the Internet headlines as he ate, and told himself that life was definitely getting better. What a thrill it would be to see Timmy running for home plate! Smith knew he might miss a few games because of work, but that was a good thing. His paycheck was secure, and if Mark Wexler's hunch was right about the future, he might see a raise before the year was over.

To make good use of the evening, he logged on to various

real estate sites and searched for apartments near the new Anzalone residence. There were several appealing choices, including one duplex with enough bedrooms to give Timmy his own room without sacrificing an office for himself. The price was more than he'd paid for the home in which he sat, which stunned him. His house had four bedrooms, three full bathrooms and a powder room, and sat on half an acre of land. The duplex was two floors with only three bedrooms, two bathrooms, and a single tiny parking space, but like Anazalone, Smith would give up one of his vehicles. Or why not get rid of them both? If ever he needed a car he could rent one.

It wasn't until after midnight that Hannah's lights panned across the front window. Smith bolted for the garage, arriving at the side of her SUV before she switched off the ignition. She put an index finger over her lips and pointed at the rear seat with her thumb. Smith eased the back door open, gently shook his son's shoulder, and then led the groggy boy into the house.

"It's not time for school, is it?" Timmy asked as he flopped onto his bed.

"You have a couple more hours," Smith told him.

"I want to play first base for the Phillies." With that, Timmy buried his head under a pillow.

Leaving his son to sleep in his clothes, Smith returned to the kitchen where Hannah stood with a glass of water. Recognizing her fatigue, he kept his tone light and his questions easy.

"I got your message," he began. "How was the drive?"

"Long," Hannah sighed. "Not much traffic, a few truck convoys."

"What did Dr. Khawaja say about Timmy?"

"The same thing as the nurse at the emergency room."

Smith was stunned. Hadn't she left a message saying Timmy

was going to be fine? Her tone had been upbeat, too, as if there was nothing to worry about. Now she was telling him that the diagnosis was the same, which wasn't a reason to celebrate.

Keeping his voice calm, he said, "Timmy has a leaking heart valve but he's going to be okay? How can that be?"

"It's late," Hannah replied. "We're both tired. Why don't we discuss this in the morning?"

Of course she was right, but Smith needed a few details so he'd be able to sleep. "Give me the short version," he said.

With a sigh, Hannah explained, "His condition does not require any drastic or immediate action. We're supposed to keep an eye on him for the next month. Another appointment is in the works, one on this side of the planet."

Her words provided genuine relief, to the point where his throat tightened and his eyes welled up. He crossed the kitchen, put his arms around Hannah, and pulled her close. "I'm so relieved," he whispered into her ear.

"They said it would be a week before we get the notice for his next appointment in the mail."

"I'll keep an eye out for it."

Hannah pulled away. "Don't forget, Timmy's not supposed to do anything strenuous. I don't want to see him riding that bike any faster than you can walk."

"Absolutely," Smith confirmed. "I guess he won't be playing in the summer league."

"No, and he's going to be bummed about that. I'm going to bed."

"I'll be right there next to you."

"We're on the same team," Ralph countered. "What's wrong with a favor for one of my own?"

"One man's favor may be another man's crime," Smith warned.

"Not the way I see it," Ralph said. "I do right by my own kind."

Smith might have agreed, albeit for different reasons, but his teammate headed up the stairs without him. His desk offered more annoyances in the form of a note from Henny Geerman and a flashing message light on his phone. Henny wanted him to stop down to her office as soon as possible. First he wanted to clear the telephone message. He cradled the receiver, entered his code, and sat up straight as Mark Wexler's recorded voice came on.

"Come up to my office first thing."

What had been a mild tension headache bloomed into a true skull-splitter. Smith found a bottle of aspirin in a drawer and swallowed two dry. Knowing his condition would not improve anytime soon, he got to his feet, grabbed a blank notepad, and headed for the stairwell.

The reception area for Mark Wexler's office featured windows looking over the oldest part of Philadelphia. While he waited, Smith gazed down at Independence Hall, the Liberty Bell Pavilion, and the Constitution Center. He couldn't remember the last time he visited these sites, but made a mental note to ask Timmy what he learned about them in his history classes.

"Mr. Wexler will see you now," the secretary said.

Smith turned from the window and headed into Wexler's sanctum.

In lieu of a desk, Wexler sat behind a broad table, which held only a telephone. This caused Smith to frown as he remembered when the same desk overflowed with heaps of blueprints and sketches.

"The governor is making Central West a first class showcase of the new stimulus bill," Wexler began. "This being Philadelphia, where the nation began and all that, he wants another ceremony with the President, the whole works. I don't have to explain one more time how important this is."

"No, sir."

"Good." After a pause, Wexler asked, "Your whole team worked with you on these revised designs and estimates, correct?"

"That's right," Smith confirmed.

"Excellent. So I don't have to worry about any surprises."

"Surprises?"

"Omissions, oversights, things that might have gone unnoticed in the rush to put it together."

"I don't think so, Mr. Wexler. If you'd like, I'll double check everything this weekend to make sure."

"What about Josh, the number two man on your team?"

"What about him?"

"He brought me the report. Does that mean he knows it as well as you?"

"He worked side by side with the rest of us. He spent a few nights on it, too. Everyone worked hard to get it done on time."

"Excellent. That gives me the confidence to soothe the governor's fears that this is one project that can come in on time and on budget."

The phone on his desk rang but Wexler only pressed a button to silence it. He looked across at Smith and began an entirely new tack.

"Henny Geerman tells me your son is having some health

issues," he said.

"He saw a specialist yesterday," Smith replied.

"She told me it's a heart problem, that she received a special notice from your Health Administration District Office."

"It can be dangerous, but for now all we can do is keep an eye on him."

"Tough break," Wexler sighed. "How are you coping?"

"Fine. It's just one of those things that happens and you have to deal with it one day at a time."

"Listen, we have the governor breathing down our neck and soon there'll be congressmen, too, and there's always city officials prancing around. That's more pressure than you may be able to handle right now."

"It's not that bad. I mean, we've been working on this project for a long time, and I have the rest of the team there to jump in if something comes up."

"I can't afford to have anything come up, Bob. This has to be flawless."

"It will be, Mr. Wexler."

"I need a guy who can keep an eye on the excavation crew every minute of the day. Then the pile drivers will be there. We can't let them do something that will make us look bad or the governor will be writing another firm's name on the check."

"Every one of us on the team has field experience, sir."

"Perfect. Then you understand that I'm forced to put Josh in as team leader until the matter of your son's health resolves itself."

"Excuse me?" Smith blurted.

"Look, it's best for everyone involved, especially you, Bob. If I had a son in this predicament, I'd be going crazy, as I'm sure you probably have over the past couple of weeks. You should have brought this to my attention."

"If I may, sir, let me explain that Timmy was to a specialist just yesterday and we're supposed to keep a close eye on him until his next appointment, which isn't due for about a month."

"According to your schedule, there's going to be a bunch of bulldozers working at Central West in a month, not to mention all the preparations between now and then."

"But ..."

Wexler put his hand up. "I know this is your baby, no pun intended, but don't be shortsighted. We all need Central West to go without a hitch. God forbid something happens to your boy, that's tragedy enough. We don't need it to snowball into a catastrophe for the rest of us."

"Honestly, Mr. Wexler, it's not that kind of thing. You would never know Timmy is anything but perfectly healthy."

Wexler shook his head. "Henny told me she has a Notice of Life Threatening Condition sitting in your file. If I don't address that what kind of person would I be? Bob, you know we look out for each other around here. It's not like I'm going to kick you to the curb."

"Are you telling me I'm off the project entirely?" Stunned that he might not be involved in something that he had literally developed from the ground up, Smith listened half-heartedly to Wexler's platitudes.

"It's what must be done. Josh can't be an effective manager if you're looking over his shoulder. Sure, you can help behind the scenes if need be but that's it. I'm going to find another spot just for you, something flexible with low stress."

All this was said with a gentle smile, with arms wide open, with all the sincerity of a visiting priest. Smith was furious. He wanted to be there when the President returned for the governor's ceremony. It was beyond unfair to deny him this honor; it was an insult. His indignation must have shown through because Wexler came around to his side of the table and put a firm hand on his shoulder.

"We're not going to leave you out," the firm's founder said. "It's just that you're going to have to watch from the sidelines for a little while. As soon as things change you'll be back in the game."

What hurt Smith most was that fighting for his job was akin to ignoring Timmy. How could he explain otherwise? All Wexler had to do was ask him what would happen if Timmy suffered an attack. In that case, Smith would be rushing to the hospital without a second thought about Central West, the governor, the President, or anything other than his son. Only a true ingrate would say otherwise.

"Are you with me?" Wexler asked.

No answer came from Smith.

"Stick with me, Bob. Who knows what this President can accomplish? Another year or two and we may be building new piers out there in the river or an extension to the airport. I'll need five guys like you."

"If all that happens you'll need a dozen," Smith croaked.

Upon hearing these words, Wexler returned to his chair. "Go see Henny," he said, pointing toward the door. "She has a program worked out for you, one that has my blessing. Whatever you need, you got it. I mean that." Then he picked up the phone and started dialing.

Smith found his way to Geerman's office, but if someone had asked him how, he would not have been able to explain the steps between Wexler's door and hers. His legs carried him along and his eyes saw people pass. None of it registered. All he could think about was that he was not going to be a part of the one project that was getting done. Someone like Ralph might have relished months of easy work and plenty of opportunity to sneak away to Ocean City or somewhere else. Not Smith. He wanted to be there from the time the first pile was driven into the mud all the way to capping the last. What was he going to tell his son now? That he was laying out curbs for a never to be built FART station? That dad had been demoted? What if the economy turned around and those piers came to fruition? He wouldn't be seen as the foundation team leader of Central West, a position he rightly held and still deserved. He would be the ditch digger on some nameless tram stop.

"Can I get you a cup of ice water?" Henny Geerman was asking.

Snapping out of his daze, Smith flopped into the chair she offered. "No, thanks. Yes. I mean, if it's not too much trouble."

"Not at all," Henny admonished him. She returned with the water, carefully handing it to Smith while she weighed his state of mind. "How did things go with Mr. Wexler?" she asked cautiously.

With a snort, Smith said, "He's taken me off Central West."

From behind a consoling look, Henny replied, "It's the best thing for you." She waited for him to say something, but after a full ten seconds, Smith uttered not a single word. He took a sip of water, stared at the glass, and shifted in his chair.

At last he asked, "Why am I here?"

"For the good news," Henny answered cheerfully. "The Universal Coverage System provides you with all kinds of support mechanisms. Mr. Wexler made it very clear that he values your contribution to the firm, and he wants you to get whatever you need during your personal crisis."

"It's not a crisis!" Smith blurted. "Timmy has a problem, but he's in school today. He's not going to drop dead any second."

The sound of those words horrified Geerman. She gripped the end of her desk, pulled herself closer to the edge, and held her gaze on Smith, trying to remember the eager young man who Mr. Wexler put on the payroll years ago. It wasn't the same person over there now. It was someone whose son was gravely ill, who lost a key position, and who was in a mild state of shock. She had been trained to deal with people facing such a situation.

"The first thing to remember," Henny began, "is that everything is temporary."

Smith considered what he'd just heard. It was true that Timmy's heart could be repaired with an operation, or it would repair itself as he grew up. Either way, as Henny had said, it was not a permanent condition.

"I suppose you're right," he admitted.

"As this unfolds, we make adjustments. You have to stay well yourself. You can't burn out worrying about Timmy or your job or anything else. You have to stay strong."

"Oh, I'm fine," Smith told her.

"I wish I had a picture of you coming through that door a few minutes ago," Henny said. "You looked like you got hit with a train."

"No, really, I'm fine. Mr. Wexler caught me off guard."

"We had a meeting yesterday afternoon about nothing but you, Bob. He truly cares. He's going to find something special for you."

"I'm glad to hear that. Maybe you can convince him to keep me on Central West."

"You'll be back there before you know it. Let me give you the rest of the good news. You've been automatically enrolled in a Wellness Support Group, which meets weekly just down the block. Your first one is tonight. Please don't miss it or the firm's Health Policy Implementation Rating will take a hit."

"You mean it's mandatory?" Smith asked. "Does my wife have to go with me?"

"In your case, a traditional family is in place. You attend the wellness meeting and your wife is available to care for Timmy. Remember, it's for your own good to learn the appropriate coping skills. And it's free, one of the many benefits of Universal Coverage."

"What about an extra gas ration? Hannah has the M Fuel Supplement Card keyed to her vehicle."

"I saw that in your file."

"In my file? How could it be in my file?"

"Not your personnel file. Your Citizen Health Profile."

"What's that?"

"Everyone has a Citizen Health Profile. It's a catch-all for your medical records and anything related to your healthcare situation. It is cross-referenced between family members and your employee file here at Wexler Associates."

"Who knew?"

"You know now," Henny said with a grin. "It's really a good system that makes sure you get the benefits you're entitled to."

"Good. So why can't I get an extra fuel ration to attend the wellness meeting."

"There's only one M Fuel Supplement Card per family. If everyone availed themselves of it, there wouldn't be enough gas to go around. The system scheduled your meeting close to your job to avoid waste."

Disappointed, Smith inquired as to what else she had in store for him.

"Mr. Wexler is looking for just the right project for you. As soon as he ..."

"You mean I don't have anything to do?" interrupted Smith.

"Job number one is taking care of Timmy."

"I'm already doing that," Smith protested. "Hannah and I are doing everything we can."

Geerman tapped her pen on her desk blotter. She admired Smith's work ethic, even wished there were more like him at the firm. Regardless, he needed to accept that now was the time to do what was really important.

"Relax. Help Josh get orientated as team leader. Take a long lunch. Maybe go for a walk through the city before your Wellness Meeting. As soon as Mr. Wexler finds a spot for you, I'll call."

"You mean I'm laid off?"

"Don't say such things!" Henny countered. "Mr. Wexler wants me to find a loophole so that you can use all your vacation days in a row. That's bending the rules, Bob. The federal mandate I told you about the last time we talked limits vacation to no more than nine consecutive days. It's part of the Keep America Working Act."

"I'm all for it, Mrs. Geerman. I want to be here doing my job."

"You will be, Bob. Keep that cell phone handy so you won't miss my call."

This is what it's like to get sacked, Smith thought. You're told to take it easy, to forget about things, to not worry. In the meantime, you go from team leader to team nobody and have all the time in the world to do things you really don't want to do.

He took a final drink of water, left the glass on Henny's desk, and turned for the door. "Thanks, Mrs. Geerman," he said.

"Hang on a second. I have to give you the details," Geerman called after him.

"Send them in an email," Smith answered over his shoulder.

The foundation team took their usual table for lunch. Smith informed them of his temporary transfer off the team and the reason for it. Given that they already knew the situation, no one was surprised, except for Josh, who seemed worried about taking the reins of such an important project.

"I'll be here to consult," Smith assured him. "Don't hesitate to ask for help."

Josh then excused himself to review their last report one more time, something he could do in the daylight outside.

The conversation shifted to the Phillies chances of making the playoffs. When this petered out, Ralph took his place on the grass for a nap and Lynn offered her usual advice.

"You should have taken your boy to the *Salvare* last week," she said to her former boss.

Not looking at his colleague, Smith said, "Why would I do that, Lynn? Timmy was just in Pittsburgh to see a specialist. He's going to be fine."

"What did that cost?"

"It didn't cost me anything. Universal Coverage has been in effect for ten years."

"I'm talking about the gas, the tolls, the wear and tear on your car," she persisted. "All that wasn't free."

"No, it wasn't," Smith said, struggling to keep his irritation under control.

"Probably cost two hundred bucks for the gas alone. The toll had to be another hundred. It's not like we don't pay twelve percent every paycheck, too."

"Please, Lynn, give me a break. I know what it cost."

"I was just saying."

"Well, let's drop it."

"Pardon me. I just want the best for Timmy. I hear that *Salvare* has facilities like you wouldn't believe."

Smith shook his head then released some of his displeasure. "Where do you hear these things, Lynn? Who tells you all this inside info about *Salvare*, because I'm not getting the same reports."

"It's around," was her reply.

"Around? Around like the rumors of Bigfoot and UFO's?"

Defiant, Lynn leaned back and stuttered a few words before coming up with a good example. "My cousin said that her friend went there for an ultrasound test that revealed a tumor in her breast."

"Good for her. I know you want to help, but every time you bring up the *Salvare* it really grates my nerves."

"I'm sorry. I didn't mean it that way."

Skipping her apology, Smith said, "Did you ever think that *Salvare* is part of the problem? Dr. Jossy and his little club of rich doctors do nothing for regular people like us. If you're super rich you can take a helicopter ride to get your hemorrhoids treated while going for a cruise to nowhere. Does that sound fair to you?"

"Not exactly, but they did find her tumor and operated the next day. She'd been waiting six months and still couldn't get an ultrasound appointment. If she hadn't gone to *Salvare*, it might have been too late the way it was for Rose. Maybe they could fix Timmy's heart in short order, and he'll be out of the woods for the rest of his life. Have you seen the commercials for that ship? The facilities look impressive."

"You should hear yourself, Lynn. You talk about *Salvare* like you're shopping for a Caribbean vacation. Is that what health-care is supposed to be about? Didn't your cousin's friend tell you about the fantastic dinner buffet or the wonderful hair salon they have on board? Oh, and while they were at it they took care of some kidney stones."

Chastised, Lynn got up from the table. "She didn't mention anything like that," she said, adding, "See you around."

Smith waited until she was out of earshot before groaning, "What a pain in the ass."

Following Henny Geerman's advice, Smith left the build-ing a few hours later. He walked to Market Street then turned left toward City Hall. The cafés cleaned up the post-lunch mess and readied for the early dinner crowd. A fair amount of people came and went from the shops. Surprised by this, he took his time, observing what was popular among the shoppers. The economy must be getting better, he thought, although nothing had improved in the suburbs. Here in the city, people were shop-ping, eating out, and generally living well. Of course they were; they didn't have to buy gasoline.

As he walked down Market Street, he thought about Joe Anzalone, who was now only a ten-minute subway ride from all of this. Smith's travel time might be half an hour, but the cost was enormous, at least forty dollars in gas and another fifty to park. If he used the FART the trip was affordable, but it could take as long as an hour and a half each way.

A few blocks on he spotted a real estate office with listings posted in the front window. Every type of living space from base-ment apartments to penthouse condominiums could be had for a price, most of which were far in excess of his mortgage, car pay-ment, and fuel bill combined. He scanned them for a two-bedroom unit that fell within his budget's range. Looking through the window he saw a young couple seated opposite one of the brokers who couldn't have been more than a year or two older than her clients. Everyone was smiling as they paged through a binder of photos. The enthusiastic broker gestured with her hands, probably extolling the virtues of an individual property the way the salesperson for Cliffwood had done.

Smith watched for a long while, entranced by the couple and their host. He recalled the nervous charge of a similar meeting, the one Hannah scheduled for a look at the house in which they currently lived. He knew they were going to buy it, as did the salesperson. And yet, the dance around the price was performed along with the inevitable concessions over free appliances and pre-paid neighborhood association fees.

"Hmmmpphh," Smith grunted in response to his own thoughts. The Cliffwood Neighborhood Association had all but dissolved. Nothing remained for the group to decide. There was no more security service to hire nor landscapers to pay nor an outfit to retain for snowplowing services. They were on their own.

Feeling dejected, he turned away from the window. Like it or not, he told himself, it was time to put the house up for sale. Anzalone was right; it didn't make sense to live in the suburbs. Smith's problem was finding a buyer. There were plenty of other homes for sale, including several in Cliffwood. He took solace in that his had been the model with all those upgrades the others lacked. He resolved to take any reasonable offer, including one on which he lost money. At least he would be free of the expensive anchor that held him away from a better standard of living.

For old time's sake, he skipped down the stairs of the Eighth Street Station of the Market Line. The train pulled in before he had a chance to marvel at the spotless station. Taking a seat, he noticed a two-year-old election poster of the President beside the system map.

"THIRD TIME'S THE CHARM," read the caption. Someone wrote, "FOUR MORE YEARS," with a black marker across the top. This was the only graffiti in the car and it was done in a legible and elegant hand.

Smith wholeheartedly agreed. The evidence of the President's success was everywhere around him. People were buying apartments. The cafés were getting ready for Friday night crowds. The subway was clean, quiet, and punctual. Above all, his son had seen a specialist and was scheduled for a follow up visit in the near future. He folded his arms, satisfied that his vote had been cast for the right man. Four more years of this President was just what the country needed, Smith thought.

He returned to daylight at 30th Street Station. Here he found crowds of people waiting for Amtrak's weekend excursion trains to Washington, D.C. and New York City. A huge banner spanned the main hall. "SAFE AND RAPID TRANSIT IS YOUR RIGHT!" it read in tall white letters on a red background. Smith wondered if this was part of the President's plan to improve intercity transit. He immediately flashed back to his earlier meeting with Mark Wexler. Maybe the next time he had a reason to go to Pittsburgh he would travel by train. Maybe those new piers would be coming soon. It made sense and he couldn't help but feel a measure of relief. His skills would be in demand like never before.

He hardly recognized the area where he and Hannah used to live. Upscale eateries, stylish boutiques, and chic houseware stores replaced the cheap Asian restaurants, coin laundries, and dive bars that Smith knew. A doorman stood in the lobby of his old building. A pair of street sweepers moved along the sidewalk with a self-propelled vacuum. They wore clean coveralls bearing clever logos and carried shiny brooms to whisk any stray debris into the throat of their machine.

Smith thought of nothing but the colossal mistake he'd made in moving to the suburbs. He should have stayed right here, trading up his living space along the way, enjoying a healthy profit each time. Instead, he'd bought the proverbial white elephant, a house that was too big and too far away. Initially, he'd enjoyed the space, especially the days in the yard with Timmy, but it had been short-sighted to remain at a fixed point in a changing world. As soon as gas prices shot up after the Second Iraq War he should have sold and moved back to the city. He might have netted a nice profit on the house, got a good deal in town, and rode the subway to work for pennies of what it cost him now. With the money he saved, he easily could have sent Timmy to an annual baseball camp.

He made up his mind to discuss the issue with Hannah as soon as possible.

While he had difficulty accepting his recent demotion, Smith could hardly bear his first Wellness Meeting. He stood in a circle of thirty people, holding hands with them in the middle of a former church, repeating what the meeting counselor, Dr. Solorzano, intoned.

"Death is part of life," Solorzano crooned.

"Death is part of life," the others said in unison.

Smith abhorred such a statement. It was inherently contradictory, akin to saying up was part of down.

"Death is part of life," came Solorzano's voice again.

"Death is part of life," replied twenty-nine voices.

Unable to say the words, Smith only moved his mouth as his eyes darted from person to person, hoping to find a like-minded soul. He was crestfallen that many of the others raised their faces toward the ceiling and called out the reply to Dr. Solorzano as if experiencing some form of rapture. The building was no longer St. Margaret's Church. Only the cornerstone bore that name as every other vestige of religious purpose had been removed. The pews in the sanctuary were gone, as were the stained glass windows, the altarpiece, and the pipe organ. Just the same, the people around Smith were in the throws of a quasi-religious experience.

"I am free of my fear of death," Dr. Solorzano said, the pitch of his voice dropping to a resonant baritone.

"I am free of my fear of death."

The point of all these chants was lost on Smith. No one gave him so much as an introduction as to how the meetings were run. He entered the building, was told to take a seat on the floor and to follow along.

Solorzano raised his hands above is head. "Death is nothing to fear."

"Death is nothing to fear."

"Now I am free."

"Now I am free."

With this phrase, Solorzano released his grip on the people next to him. "Embrace the person next to you and express your sense of relief."

Not knowing what to do, Smith stood awkwardly among the others. He suddenly found himself in the clutches of a sweaty man who squeezed him hard enough to force the air out of his lungs.

"I feel so much better," the man said. "I'm not afraid. I'm ready to move on. How about you?"

"I don't know," Smith replied, which was true. He had no

idea how he was supposed to feel.

"Don't hold back," the man advised. "I held back for two months. Then Missy took a turn for the worse. I could hardly take it. Now that I've set myself free of the fear, I'm happy, healthy, strong. You know?"

"What about ... uh ... Missy?"

"She's hanging on. They say she has another month or so before it's over."

"Over?" Smith echoed.

"You can't say it, can you? Death. You can't say the word."

"Sure I can. I was being polite."

"You're new. You have to let go. You have to listen to Dr. Solorzano. You have to accept that death is part of life and then the discomfort will leave you. Don't hold back."

This is crazy, Smith thought, heading for the door.

Before he could find his way out, Dr. Solorzano addressed him directly. "Tell us your name and why you're here," he said.

It took Smith a few seconds to realize that everyone awaited his reply. He wished he could make himself disappear. Since he wasn't a magician, he said, "My name is Bob Smith. I'm here because ... because ... well, because I have to be or ..."

"We're all here because we need to be here," Solorzano interjected. "We need solace. We need comfort. We need to know that we're going to be okay even if someone else in our life will not. Isn't that true for you?"

"Not exactly," Smith replied.

"Please, don't make a struggle of it. Tell us your tragedy. The sooner you face death, the sooner you'll be free."

Again, Smith wanted to melt into a crack in the floor. Had he been in the presence of a Wexler client, even the governor or the President of the United States, he could have explained without fear exactly how the foundation of Central West was to be built. He could have done that without a drop of sweat on his brow. Amidst these strangers, in this odd place, sitting on the floor instead of a comfortable chair, he was out of his element.

"Is your wife terminal?" Solorzano asked.

"No."

"Your father?"

"No."

"Who?"

"No one."

"No one?" Solorzano scoffed. "We're all terminal. We're all going to die. Oh, forgive me, maybe you're some kind immortal, like a comic book hero." This elicited a laugh from the group. "Let me make this easy. Is anyone close to you ill?"

"My son, Timmy."

"Explain," Solorzano beamed.

"He's not going to die or anything," Smith continued.

"Let me stop you there. We're all going to die. Let me hear you say it."

"Timmy's not going to die. He's only eleven."

Shaking his head, Solorzano said, "You have a long way to go Robert Smith."

It was an interminable meeting, lasting more than two hours. Smith finally gave in to Solorzano's cajoling. He explained Timmy's problem, admitted that his son might die, and that he himself would also die. Stating these obvious facts aloud in front of strangers gave him no peace. If anything he was disconcerted by the whole affair. He rebuffed entreaties by a pair of attendees who wanted him to join them for a post-meeting drink. He'd rather gulp boilermakers with the crew of a pile-driving rig than spend another minute with these people.

So out of sorts was he that he pondered calling Hannah to pick him up. In the end, he rejected the idea because she had a girl's night out tomorrow. If she collected him in the city she wouldn't have the gas to meet her friends. He preferred not to inconvenience her, especially for something like this. He might pay for it in unforeseeable ways. Therefore, he walked to the subway, used his newly minted pass, and took a seat on the first westbound train.

As the car filled, Smith's jitters abated. All around him, the Friday evening revelers took their positions. The women scented with perfume, the men wearing glittering watches, and both sexes smartly dressed, they teemed like a school of shiny fish in an undersized tank. Their energy enthused Smith, giving him the boost he needed to regain his poise. His life wasn't much different than these people. For the moment, he was stuck on the outside, in the distant suburbs and in a holding pattern career-wise. No matter. He discovered his mistakes and was on his way to correcting them. In no time, a year at most, he would be side by side with Hannah, on the way to a show or a dinner out, probably riding this exact car, exchanging the same knowing glances as this crowd. He'd be looking for that last nanny Timmy had, the young woman from Poland. What was her name? Nadzia. Yes, he would need Nadzia to keep an eye on Timmy while he and Hannah were out on the town. And he would have the money to pay for it all thanks to the new projects Mark Wexler had talked about.

He held his briefcase atop his lap, saw another poster of the President on the wall through the window, and read the tag line.

"ONE FOR ALL."

"One," Smith said to himself, "One for all." He was thinking of himself, Hannah, and Timmy. They were going to be part of this set, the people who lived well, enjoyed life, and had no regrets.

"DEATH CAN BE VERY EDUCATIONAL."

CHAPTER ELEVEN

AMERICA SERVES AMERICA published regional volunteer opportunity guides each month. They arrived in every mailbox regardless of the recipient's desire to participate. Glossy pages covered with handsome photos showed young people working together with their fellow citizens as part of their monthly service. Everyone smiled whether they pulled rakes across a city park or pushed a wheelchair-bound person through the halls of a nursing home. Some advertised opportunities offered compensation, which varied depending upon the level of commitment required. Certain positions offered tax breaks, others granted fuel vouchers, and a few awarded college credit.

Smith took his time going through the ASA guide. He

stopped on a page where the City of Philadelphia sought people to assist with a cleanup along the Schuylkill River. He wasn't as interested in the job as he was in the fuel voucher it offered: 10 gallons for 32 hours served. He might also network with Philadelphia residents and learn first-hand details about neighborhoods, available apartments, and the local scene.

After marking the page, Smith continued his search. There were a few more opportunities that appealed to him, either for the compensation, contacts, or actual job to be done. Although, when he figured his cost of getting to and from them, most yielded a marginal return at best. In some instances, he was worse off than if he did nothing. What bugged him most was that there was none available anywhere beyond the city's borders. It chafed his acknowledged error of leaving the city.

Setting the booklet aside, Smith reconsidered Doctor Ben's offer. It was close by and it paid cash. Tucking his tail was a small price to pay in light of what could be gained. Just the same, he didn't want to get involved in something that violated numerous environmental statutes.

Hannah joined him at the breakfast table, saw the ASA guide, and gave him a quizzical look. A lousy liar, Smith thought it best to tell her about his temporary furlough, but not before revealing his plan to move into the city. She needed no convincing, stating unequivocally that she was ready to leave Cliffwood at a moment's notice. She was worried about their financial position and this provided Smith with the opening to bring up what happened the day before at work.

"I'm just glad they didn't fire you," she said after he told her he'd been transferred off Central West. "We'd be in real trouble if that happened."

"Wexler can't," Smith said confidently. "Henny Geerman

gave me that line about my vacation days, but the Universal Coverage Manual has an entire section on employer responsibilities. I double-checked it early this morning and six months paid leave without fear of losing my job is the iron-clad law of the land."

"You're not the team leader anymore, and you're not working on anything else," Hannah put in. "So you kind of did lose it."

As he read through the section in the UC Manual this reality occurred to Smith. He considered taking it up with Henny Geerman, and if that didn't work, with Mark Wexler, but then thought better of the idea. Yes, Central West was an important project. Nonetheless, the bigger picture was his own future, and if he really wanted to get ahead in life, he had to leave the suburbs. The only way to free himself from Cliffwood was to make some extra money so that he could afford the move. Their combined salaries paid the bills but nothing remained to be saved. A side job, preferably one close to home, was the obvious solution and he revealed the previous week's visit to Doctor Ben in that light.

"I don't know about that guy," Hannah said when Smith told her Ben had offered him work at the Thorpe Estate. "Weren't there some kind of militia meetings out there a few years back? A bunch of gun nuts or something?"

"No, that was in Schuylkill County," Smith replied, then added, "Doctor Ben has some old buildings. He's restoring them to their original condition."

"It sounds like a job for a regular contractor," Hannah said.

She was right and Smith told her so. "At the same time," he added, "If we want to get out of here, I need to make some extra money. Maybe I'll take those vacation days after all and moonlight with ASA."

"Timmy's going to miss you at his games," Hannah reminded her husband.

Taking a line from Henny Geerman, he said, "It's only temporary. Think of all the stuff we can do together in the city."

"That's true," Hannah agreed then asked, "Aren't you double dipping by taking paid vacation then grabbing gas rations or supplemental pay? ASA was designed for unemployed people, honey, people who are really down on their luck."

"Yeah," Smith admitted.

"Why don't you wait a few weeks, maybe until after Timmy's next appointment? If things work out, you'll be team leader again and everything will be back to normal."

She was asking him to tread water for a month, perhaps longer, but he didn't want to be a thief of sorts by taking advantage of the ASA program benefits when they might go further for someone else in need.

"It's not like we're living in the street," Hannah said. "Look at this house."

Smith had seen enough of their house. It was almost a Mc-Mansion, the kind of house he and Hannah criticized during their early college days. It was comfortable, or rather, it had been comfortable when gas was only three dollars a gallon. The cocktail and dinner parties, the visiting family stay-overs, and private spaces had been enjoyed by each of them. Nonetheless, Smith wondered how he and his family had become part of the problem when they had rallied for all the solutions.

Before he could answer the question, Timmy entered the room.

"Hey champ," Smith said. "I hear you didn't do well on your math test."

"I don't want to keep the stats for the team," Timmy replied. "I want to play."

"That's no excuse for getting a D on your exam," Smith countered.

"I'll do better next time."

"You have to do better every time."

"How am I gonna do that without batting practice?"

Hannah said, "Your father is talking about your math test."

Timmy's slump continued through the final weeks of the school year. His streak of straight A's fell in the final marking period when two B's appeared on his last report card. He refused to keep statistics for his team, going so far as to ignore a personal plea from Mr. Dolante, the Moguls' coach. He was a player and belonged on the field. Besides, Bev Stong kept the statistics. How would he look sitting next to a girl with a pencil in his hand as opposed to tapping a bat on home plate before the next pitch?

Hannah wanted to take him to a psychiatrist, a move Smith felt would only further damage the boy's self image. The real solution was to get his heart condition rectified so that he could get out on the field and win.

Luckily for Smith, Timmy's appointment notice hung on the refrigerator. It came on the same day as his new Universal Coverage Card.

Unbeknownst to his father, Timmy kept a calender under his bed. He marked off the days until the appointment. He lay awake at night, imagining what he would tell the doctor.

"I'm the fastest kid on the team. I stole more bases than anyone."

The doctor would nod his head at this, and say, "I bet you are Timmy. I listened to your heart and it sounds fine. Get out there and win!"

Then he would have to play catch up with the Media Moguls, whose summer season had just begun. He saw himself in the batting cage, smacking fast pitches from Mr. Dolante. He envisioned the Moguls making the trip to Philadelphia for a game against Joey Anzalone's team, a challenge arranged by Timmy himself to settle a grudge. Joey had been his pal, but in the weeks since he left Cliffwood, Timmy hadn't heard from him. That put him on the other team, which was synonymous with being a loser because the Moguls were on the way to a championship with or without a great outfielder. The other kids would have to fill the gap.

The week before his appointment, Timmy perked up. He sat on the couch with his glove and ball, watching the Phillies on ESPN. Inspired by the pros, he fantasized about his own future in the game. He liked the nostalgia uniforms with their pinstripes and the stylized P on the caps. His mom smiled when he asked for the complete outfit for Christmas.

"Get straight A's and you'll find one under the tree," she told him.

Straight A's are easy, Timmy wanted to tell her. The only reason he got those two B's was because he messed up a couple of final exams. He was upset about not being in the game, but he was back on track now that the summer semester was underway. It was mostly review, anyway, a chance for the dumb kids to catch up. He wasn't dumb and he knew it. Mr. Dolante told him that if he earned good grades and played like a champion he could become a Scholar Athlete in high school. Scholar Athletes received money from colleges with top baseball teams.

"If you want to play in the majors," Mr. Dolante said, "You have to come out of a program like that. You have to start early if you want to get in."

In other words, catching up was difficult, which is why he was so upset about missing practice and the start of the season. He studiously watched the pros play and mimicked their moves when no one was around. There had been a guy named Schmidt who played for the Phillies, but the current roster listed not one Smith. Thus, there was room for him to live up to the big guy's legacy.

Like his son, Bob Smith spent the better part of a month doing nothing important. He burned some of his vacation time by taking three consecutive Mondays off. Against Mark Wexler's orders, he peeked in at Central West where the primary excavation crew cleared the site in preparation for the first shovel ceremony. He watched a bulldozer grade the spot where soon pile-driving rigs would arrange themselves.

He didn't need a calendar to mark the days. His wellness meetings paced the month for him, and as the fourth one began, he found himself seated opposite Leslie, a woman in her mid-fifties who reminded him of his mother when he was Timmy's age. They were supposed to practice telling a family member about the death of a spouse. After going through the rudiments prescribed by Dr. Solorzano both Smith and Leslie turned to other topics.

Smith told her about Timmy's appointment on the coming Monday.

"You're lucky to be on a CGP," Leslie said, "My husband worked for a plumbing supply house. He was number one thirty six on the chemo roster."

"I'm sorry to hear that," Smith said, interpreting her reference in the past tense to mean her husband had already died despite the fact she seemed too upbeat for someone who had recently lost her life partner.

"There's no reason to be sorry," Leslie said with a wave of her hand. "Phil is fine."

"Oh, good," Smith put in, and after a pause added, "I'm glad to hear he got the treatment he needed."

"He got it all right," she said, then stole a glance around the room to see if anyone had heard her. "Let me tell you the story," she continued. "He had a lump in his neck that didn't go away. I made an appointment for him through the HAO. He finally got in two months later and the doctor pegged his problem right away. It was Hodgkin's Lymphoma."

Smith nodded that he was familiar with the disease in a cursory way.

"The doctor said as long as he got chemo right away he had a ninety percent chance of a complete recovery."

"I've heard that," Smith said, "and it sounds like it worked out for him."

"Not exactly. The Health Administration District Office in Bucks County — that's where we live — wanted more details from the doctor, something about the stage of Phil's cancer. Whatever. To get back in to see the doctor was going to be another month, maybe longer." Leslie paused for another look around the room. Other pairs of attendees were busy hugging, weeping, and explaining their less hopeful situations. Finally, she said, "I admit that I panicked. What were we supposed to do? Hodgkins is curable, if you don't fool around. You have to get treatment right away. What would anyone do in that situation?"

Empathizing with Leslie's feelings, Smith said, "I'm sure you did the right thing."

"I think I did," Leslie replied. "I got in touch with the *Salvare*."

"You're kidding," Smith blurted.

Sensing that she might have trusted the wrong person, Leslie looked over her shoulder then back at Smith. "It's over now, so it doesn't matter," she finished.

"Then why are you here?" asked Smith.

"These meetings are mandatory until your family member either dies or you are released."

"How do you get released?"

"When the diagnosis changes. As soon as Phil gets in at the clinic, I'll be finished with this. That is if the Care Delivery Specialist does the paperwork right."

Dr. Solorzano crossed the room to Smith and Leslie. "How are we coping this evening?" he wanted to know.

"Good," Leslie answered.

"How about you, Mr. Smith?"

Confused was the answer Smith wanted to give. How could he blame Leslie for going to the *Salvare*? If caught in time, her husband's disease was easily cured. Certainly, no one would have deliberately made her husband wait for treatment if his life was in danger. Who could be so callous? She should have stuck to the system, which would have given her husband everything he needed after a minor delay. His own experience with Timmy proved his point. But she panicked, and while it turned out alright, it must have cost her a bundle.

"Learning," Smith said to Dr. Solorzano, who was waiting for an answer.

"Death can be very educational," Solorzano told him.

"OKAY. HOW ABOUT THE REST OF YOU? ANY CHEST PAIN?"

CHAPTER TWELVE

TIMMY WAITED JUST INSIDE THE DOOR with both hands on the panic bar. He wanted to get the doctor's appointment over with to put this trouble with his heart behind him forever. After the appointment, he planned on taking his place as shortstop that afternoon. He had his glove, uniform, and cleats in his knapsack to save his dad the trouble and gas of going home first.

As Smith rounded the corner into the parking lot at Media North Elementary School, he saw his son dart from the building. In a flash the boy had the passenger door open and hopped onto the seat like a bank robber, or an eleven-year-old headed for home plate.

"Let's go dad," Timmy urged.

"Always look both ways before you pull out," Smith reminded his son. "That goes for crossing the street, too."

"I know."

This was Smith's fourth Monday off in a row. At least this one had a purpose, taking Timmy to his follow up appointment at the Adler Cardiac Clinic in Philadelphia. Thanks to the M Fuel Supplement card, he had plenty of fuel to make the trip, the only catch being that he had to siphon it from Hannah's SUV into his pickup because the card was keyed to her license plate. It wasn't his first time using the siphon. During the previous four weeks, he gradually filled the two five gallon jugs in the garage. In the event of another emergency, he would have plenty of gas to get to the hospital. He meant to tell Hannah about it but never found the right moment. She would probably just think him paranoid.

Which left him in the left seat with his son on the other side of the pickup, feeling less paranoid than simply fearful. As much as Smith admired his son's optimism, he feared what the next doctor might say. It was unrealistic to expect that Timmy's heart had fixed itself already. It was equally unlikely that the first two doctors had mistakenly diagnosed the problem.

"I ate a big lunch today," Timmy said out of the blue.

"Good," Smith replied, knowing the reason. "Let's not get ahead of ourselves."

"I'm not worried, dad. I feel great. I'm ready to play."

Cautiously, Smith advised, "We'll see if the doctor agrees."

Located on Temple University's campus, Smith found the Adler Cardiac Clinic with no trouble. He tucked his receipt for the forty dollar parking fee into his jacket with the hope that he could deduct the expense from his income taxes. He would have to check the Universal Coverage Manual later because Timmy was already out of the truck and striding for the door.

Catching up, Smith nearly dumped Timmy's records out of the folder he made for them. "Slow down. You're not on the field yet," he said as they entered the clinic.

Inside, father and son passed through an airport-style metal detector. Two guards sporting none of the corrupt jocularity of Rieser monitored the line while another pair searched septuagenarians and younger souls with equal vigor.

"Why do they have cops here?" Timmy asked a little too loud for his dad's comfort.

"To keep us safe," Smith answered, shepherding his son toward the next line, which ended at the reception window. After a brief wait, he received a yellow plastic tag bearing the letter C and was told to take a seat until he was called.

"Let's put the game on," Timmy urged, referring to the television mounted on the far wall.

"There were other people here before you."

"Maybe they're Phillies fans, too."

Resisting a smile at his son's wit, Smith said, "Sit tight. It won't be long. Next time bring one of your school books."

"There won't be a next time," Timmy said more to himself than his father.

Looking about the room, Smith noticed several other yellow tags. Green, red, and blue ones were also scattered among the fifty or so people in the waiting room.

A thin man wearing a T-shirt over faded blue jeans entered the room carrying a clipboard. "Group C," he called. "Everyone in Group C follow me."

"That's us, dad," Timmy said and leapt to his feet.

"Be careful," Smith warned, catching Timmy's arm before he bowled into an elderly man with a walker.

"Sorry, mister," Timmy said to him.

"Fall in behind me, young man."

Foiled in his hurry, Timmy shuffled along, aware that his dad was glaring at him.

The group entered a smaller room containing a row of fifteen chairs, one for each patient, but not enough for those accompanying them. Three more faced the row from behind a steel desk. Timmy rushed for one of the seats but made it only a few feet before Smith pulled him back.

"Look, Timmy, I know you're in a hurry, but don't be rude. Your mother and I raised you better than that. There are people here old enough to be your grandfather. The right thing to do is to give someone a seat who needs it more than you."

"But I'm ..."

"Timmy," Smith said in a tone that his son knew better than to challenge.

The fellow with the clipboard surveyed the group for a few moments before asking everyone to hold up their yellow tag. "For those of you who haven't done this before," he said, "My name is Clark Faber. I'm the Care Delivery Specialist who will be overseeing your visit today with Dr. Hillman. Any questions you may have regarding the delivery of the care you receive today should be directed to me. I'm going to ask some questions. Please answer them concisely and directly. After I've completed a general review, you will be seen by the doctor." With that he took one of the three chairs that faced the group.

"I knew he was going to say that," Timmy said.

"Shhh," Smith whispered to his son.

"Raise your hand if you have experienced any acute symptoms since your last visit." Faber began.

The man with the walker raised his hand.

"What kind of acute symptoms?"

"Pain, right here," came the answer with a hand across his chest.

"How would you rate the pain?"

"I don't know. It hurt."

No one reacted, but Smith sensed there might be a burst of laughter. He hoped Timmy didn't start it.

"It hurt," Faber repeated. "On a scale of one to ten, how would you rate your pain?"

"It hurt is all I can say."

"Okay. How about the rest of you? Any chest pain?"

"A little," someone called out.

Faber shook his head. "Be specific."

"Three," the same person said.

"That's better. Three on the ten scale. Please people, now is the time to help me order the care sequence. Any more symptoms?"

Gradually, the people in the room related how they felt. Faber had to brush off an obese guy who went on for several minutes about his experience climbing the stairs to his apartment during an Energy Conservation Event. If not, the description might have lasted fifteen minutes.

Through all this Timmy sat quietly, fidgeting now and then, but nothing worse, which impressed Smith. Although his son was generally a well-behaved boy, it was a lot to expect him to sit through these medical histories, especially on a game day. Smith himself didn't quite understand what was going on. Clearly Faber wasn't a doctor. At any rate, he was playing part of the role by listening to the patients. He took their names, noted their comments, and arranged his files accordingly.

Before Smith could figure out the system, Dr. Hillman entered the room. He wore the white coat and stethoscope of a physician, along with the harried demeanor of someone with too much to do. He addressed the group in a languid voice, saying, "Time for cardiac review, everyone."

No one responded as the doctor sat down next to Faber, which left only one chair unoccupied. Then a woman rose off her chair, strode forward, and pulled off her shirt. "I can see my file on top," she said. "Let's get this over with doc."

Timmy gawked at the shirtless woman who moved to the front of the room. She put herself in the last empty chair with all the finesse of a truck driver then dropped her appointment slip and tag on Faber's lap.

"Do me a favor and don't stare," she said to him. "I'm old enough to be your grandmother."

Straightening up, Faber made a production of reviewing her paperwork while Dr. Hillman put his stethoscope to her chest.

Shocked by the scene before him, Smith stood up and headed for the door, intent on rectifying what had to be a mistake. Timmy's appointment memorandum said nothing about a group setting. It must have been mixed up with a general evaluation of some sort. He wasn't going to have his son staring at an old woman's breasts.

"Please remain on the other side of the room until you are called or the session has ended," Faber ordered Smith.

"I think I'm in the wrong place," Smith replied.

"You have a yellow tag, don't you?"

"Yes," Smith said, fingering the chip in his hand.

"Then you're in the right place. Be patient until I call your name."

"Can I have a word with you in private?"

"This is as private as it gets at this level," Faber replied.

"Does Timmy's heart have the kind of problem that may come and go? Maybe the valve works correctly sometimes and other times it doesn't."

"I don't think so. The heart is like any other type of plumbing. Once it starts to leak it rarely gets better without some work by the plumber."

"So then what caused Timmy to collapse on the field?"

"Could have been one of many things. Overexertion is the simplest explanation but not necessarily the correct one."

"Right on," Timmy whispered without looking up at this dad.

"Why would those other doctors have said it's a valve problem when it's not?" Smith asked next.

"Incompetence?" Hillman shrugged.

Faber pointed his pen at the doctor and warned, "That statement has no basis in fact."

"It was a question, not a statement."

"Dr. Hillman, you risk an official sanction if you do not retract the comment."

Looking at Smith, Hillman said, "I have no idea why someone I don't know might have given one diagnosis or the other. All I can say is they would not have graduated from the same medical school I did. Maybe the standards have changed."

Annoyed, Faber shoved his completed form in front of the doctor for a signature. After getting it, he tore off the top copy then separated the other two. These he stuffed into separate files and finally slapped the last one on top of the folder Smith used for all of Timmy's records.

"You're free to go," he said.

"Wait a minute," Smith said. "Is Timmy going to be okay?"

"If I were still in private practice …" Hillman replied before Faber cut him off again.

"Dr. Hillman, you are an independent contractor employed by the Universal Coverage System. Please don't mislead the client."

"I'm talking to the kid's dad," Hillman fired back, "and I was going to tell him that in the past I would make some other recommendations, tests and so forth to help pinpoint the problem."

"You're speculating," Faber said.

"I certainly am. That's why we have tests: to determine whether our speculation is right or wrong."

"Which can be a waste of resources that only creates unnecessary anxiety in the patient."

"Who's doing the speculating?"

"I just want to know if Timmy's going to be okay," Smith put in.

Hillman stood up, put his hand on the boy's shoulder, and asked, "What position do you play?"

"Shortstop," Timmy said brightly.

"My son was a second baseman," Hillman said. "I think you're well enough to play your position, but do your dad a favor."

"Sure, what?"

"If you don't feel good, tell him right away. Maybe you feel a little dizzy or lightheaded or weak. You could have some pain in your chest or your arm. Things like that. Don't keep going. Stop. You tell your dad and he'll get you some help. Get to a doctor immediately. Can you do that for me?"

"I can," Timmy assured him.

"Good. Keep your eye on the ball."

This was the kind of thing Smith expected from a doctor. It wasn't exactly a clean bill of health, but it was a frank explanation. Unfortunately, none of the medical professionals he met to this point had been as forthcoming. He couldn't imagine why. It was their job.

"Thank you, doctor," Smith said. "Can you tell me what kind of tests I should get?"

"The short answer is to start with an ECG stress test because Timmy suffered an attack while engaged in physical activity. This may pick up a problem with the heart's electrical system for lack of a better term. If that doesn't show anything, the next step would be a Holter Monitor for several days to record the heart's activity over a longer period."

"Do you think the problem is related to the electrical system as you put it?" Smith asked.

Hillman replied, "It could be arrhythmia, which is tricky. Sometimes the heart beats too fast or two slow or the chambers get out of synch. I can't say for sure without the tests."

"How do I arrange those?" Smith asked.

Dr. Hillman cocked his head toward Faber.

"How do I arrange those tests?" Smith repeated to the CDS.

"Schedule an appointment through your Health Admin Office," Faber answered.

Recalling his previous experience at that office, Smith requested whatever paperwork might be necessary to secure such an appointment.

Faber said, "You already have everything you need."

"Are you sure?"

"Are you asking me if I know how to do my job?"

Keeping his cool, Smith said, "I'm asking if I need a referral or authorization of some kind, which is what was required for the second opinion."

"And my answer is the same."

Finished with the bureaucrat, Smith turned his attention back to Dr. Hillman. "Do you think it's wise for Timmy to go about normal activities like baseball and phys-ed at school?"

"I'd like to see those test results," Hillman said. "Until then, as long as everyone is aware of what to do in the event of an emergency, he should be okay."

It was the kind of answer Smith might have given in his own field. He wouldn't tell a developer how tall a building could be built without first knowing the specifics of the ground it was to be built upon. The public had been told the residential towers at Central West were going to be more than twenty stories before the soil analysis was complete. The President's speech was meant to be inspirational and a difference of five stories, or even ten, was something that could be worked out later. Did Smith have the same latitude with his son's life?

"Are you going to let your dad know if you don't feel well?" Hillman asked Timmy.

"I will. I promise," Timmy answered.

"Good luck on the field, and don't let your dad down."

The crack from Timmy's bat had the crowd on their feet. The ball flew straight over the pitcher's head, soared across the outfield, and landed somewhere behind the centerfield wall. It was only the third pitch to Timmy, the first two being a strike and a ball that he allowed to pass without even twitching. As the third one came in, he stepped into his swing, leveling the bat across its path until contact was made. He didn't stop there the way some kids did. He followed through, all the way to the point where the tip of the bat hung high above and behind his right shoulder. He didn't have to look for the ball. He knew it was gone.

The crowd rewarded him with their cheers. Mr. Dolante smacked his butt as he rounded first base. He jogged around the diamond, tapping home plate with a toe before retreating to the dugout. He wanted to wave to his dad, but that would have been silly. He knew his dad worried too much about him. Didn't he just hit a home run after a month without practicing? And if Dr. Hillman asked him how he felt as he slapped hands with his teammates, he would have said that he never felt better. I swear, Timmy said to himself, I'm ready for the World Series.

"That kid of yours is a natural," Mr. Dolante said to Smith. "Amazing."

"Thanks, coach," Smith replied. Allowing Timmy to play was the hardest decision he'd made in his life. No sooner were they in the truck than Timmy wanted to change into his uniform. It was a standoff between father and son for the first ten minutes of the drive. Smith didn't want to deny his son the thrill of playing nor did he want him to collapse on the field again.

As they merged onto the Interstate, Smith weighed what the doctor said with his desire to make Timmy happy. In the end he made a deal with himself. He would let Timmy play but also request the tests Dr. Hillman recommended. Plus, he would keep a close eye on his son, especially at his games.

Entering the Borough of Media, they saw Mr. Fetterman walking toward the field, which was located just at the edge of town. They pulled over and offered him a ride.

"That uniform hasn't seen a grass stain in quite a while," commented Fetterman.

"It will today," Timmy confirmed.

"If I was still a tailor, I'd make the whole team snazzy new outfits."

"Like the one's the Phillies wore last month?"

"How about like the one I'm wearing now?" Fetterman asked.

"This was mine in high school."

With Timmy's help, the Media Moguls won the game handily, thereby breaking a four-game losing streak. Coach Dolante gave the boys a pep talk about teamwork, practice, and sportsmanship that reminded Smith of the President's speech at Central West.

"One for all" was not only a catch phrase; it was a way of life, one that Smith fully embraced. Whether on the baseball field or a construction site or a nation for that matter, everyone had to work together. He was looking forward to getting back on the team and in the game.

"TODAY IS MY BIRTHDAY, MR. SMITH, NOT YOURS."

CHAPTER
THIRTEEN

SEVERAL DAYS AFTER TIMMY TOOK TO THE FIELD, Smith searched his home office for the family's digital camera. After not finding it, he asked Hannah if she knew where it was.

"Look in the drawer by the fridge," she answered.

There it was, in its case where it belonged, but with a dead battery. He connected the charger and plugged it into an outlet above the kitchen counter.

"Are you coming to this afternoon's game?" Timmy asked from over his cereal bowl. "It doesn't start until six."

"I have my meeting tonight," Smith told his son, referring to the two hours he was obligated to spend in Dr. Solorzano's company. He would have preferred to be at Timmy's game, but there was no escaping the wellness meeting. He'd presented Henny Geerman with Timmy's new diagnosis as signed by Dr. Hillman, but it wasn't enough to free him from this Universal Coverage requirement. Similarly, he couldn't return to his position as team leader.

"As soon as the paperwork catches up," Henny had explained, "I'll let you know."

"Thanks, Mrs. Geerman. I'd like to be there for the first shovel ceremony," Smith said.

"Let me check the schedule," she replied.

Knowing the date, Smith said, "It's next Thursday."

"Oh, the computers will be in synch by then," Henny promised him and followed up with a firm reminder that he not miss his group session with Dr. Solorzano.

Thus, the only thing on Smith's Friday schedule was a trip to the Health Administration District Office followed by the wellness meeting. He planned to snap a few shots of Rieser and Plant retrieving their bribes from under that cement block. Without a full battery, he was out of luck. He thought about using the camera on his cell phone, but the resolution wasn't very good. He wanted clear images of the money, the men picking it up, and then people going to the head of the line. He wasn't sure what he was going to do with them; he would figure that out later. It was his duty as an honest citizen to expose this kind of corruption. If not, how would the authorities know?

"Good luck at the game," Smith said to Timmy as he left the house.

Another vacation day down the drain, Smith thought as he drove to the HAO, burning gas that would have been better used taking him to Timmy's game. He rode the FART every day to conserve his fuel ration. He had nothing important to do for

Wexler Associates, so it didn't matter if the train was early or late, though it typically pulled in half an hour or more after the scheduled time.

Arriving at HAO 117, Smith debated whether or not he was going to pay the fifty-dollar bribe to get ahead in the line. He decided against it for two reasons. In the first place, money only perpetuated the problem. Secondly, fifty dollars was not pocket change. He took his place early, among several dozen others who were either unaware of Rieser's system or lacked the money to participate.

To his surprise, Mr. Fetterman showed up a few minutes later.

"Your boy plays a heck of a game," the retired tailor said.

"Thanks."

"What are you doing back here?"

"Scheduling some follow-up tests for Timmy. How about you?"

"I need a prescription renewal. Before all these machinations, I used to just call my doctor and he'd let the pharmacy know to renew it. Now I have to come here and get approval, then take that to Dispensary 22, which wouldn't be so bad, but I have to ride the bus and change lines. Sometimes I get stuck at the middle stop and then just go home because 22 will close before I get there."

"Maybe they could give you three months at one time and save you the trouble."

"Hah! They don't have three months worth of stock," Fetterman countered. "One time I went there and the lady pushing the pills told me she could only give me seven, enough for a week. The way the buses run in this county I was lucky to get back there in time to fill the rest of the prescription on the day I took the last one."

"I'm sure it was just a glitch in the system, what we call a supply chain error," Smith said, using jargon he knew well. "Better than having an insurance company cut you off."

Rolling his eyes, Fetterman remarked, "You're starting to sound like one of them."

"In the end you got your medication," Smith reminded him.

"Yeah, Doctor Ben does what he can, too. He's the only one who gives a damn. The rest of this bunch, they just see me as one old man in line with all the others, someone waiting for an I double-E."

"I double-E?" Smith asked.

"Lattner! Forsman! Peters!" Rieser called before Smith's question was answered. More names followed until several of them got into a shoving match at the door.

"Knock it off!" Rieser hollered. When two people refused to stop, he strode up to them, grabbed each by the arm like children and dragged them to the back of the line.

"Guess they're stuck here like the rest of us," Fetterman said.

Nodding, Smith couldn't help but take a small measure of satisfaction in their fate. They broke the rules and their continued impatience only led to the severe enforcement of them. In the process, their fifty-dollar bribe became a fine, and Smith was two places closer to speaking with a Care Administration Specialist.

He waited until after lunch for his number to flash on the screen. He found himself seated before Ms. Buckley again, the woman who had challenged him over Timmy's second opinion in Pittsburgh. As he sat down beside her desk, Smith carefully gauged her mood. He didn't want a problem now that Timmy was back on track.

"Let's see here," Buckley said as she looked over Timmy's file.

Smith took her friendly tone to mean that she either didn't remember him or wasn't holding a grudge. Given the number of people who passed through the HAO it was probably the former. Either way, he took it for what it was worth: a good sign that he might get what he wanted.

"It seems Timmy has been for a second opinion and then had a cardiac review just a few days ago," Buckley continued. "What can I do for you today, Mr. Smith?"

"I'd like to schedule an ECG stress test," he said. "Dr. Hillman ..."

"Well, would you look at this!" cheered Buckley, clapping her hands and looking past Smith to a group of her colleagues who wheeled a cart laden with a birthday cake down the aisle.

"Happy Birthday to you. Happy Birthday to you," they sang. "Happy Birthday dear Olga. Happy Birthday to you!"

Buckley leaned over the cake, blew out the candles, and then hugged each of her co-workers. The cake was cut, the pieces handed out, and a carafe of coffee used to refill everyone's mug. While Smith and several other clients waited, the group enjoyed their party. They spent the better part of an hour, enough time for Smith to need the men's room. He darted in and out, afraid that if he failed to return before Buckley, he might lose his spot to someone else.

He worried for nothing, because Buckley flopped into her chair with a smudge of blue icing on her face and the same genial attitude with which she had greeted him earlier.

"How nice of them, don't you think?" she said to Smith.

He agreed that it was a pleasant gesture without mentioning that the timing could have been better. Couldn't they have had the cake during their lunch break? The candles would have shone so much brighter during the lights out period of the Energy Conservation Event.

"Where were we?" Buckley asked herself as she shuffled through Timmy's paperwork. "Oh, yes, here's my note, an ECG Stress Test is what you were looking for."

"For my son," Smith said.

"Right," Buckley drawled as she tapped at her keyboard. She stopped abruptly, looked over at Smith and said, "Let me have your referral."

"Uh ..." Smith stuttered. "I was told I had everything thing I needed."

"You can't expect me to schedule an advanced test without a referral. That's the minimum. By rights you should have a prescription from a cardiologist co-signed by the Care Delivery Specialist."

"The CDS told me I had everything I needed," Smith snapped.

"The system changed six months ago, and the CDS might have been in the second training group, which means he wouldn't know that advanced tests require co-signed referrals and/or a similarly endorsed prescription in order to be authorized."

Clark Faber, for all his haughtiness wasn't even aware of changes in the system he was supposed to supervise. While the fault lay with Faber, Smith was the victim. He spent more than half his day, suffered through an impromptu birthday party, and nearly burst his bladder waiting to discover this fact. The worst part was that there was nothing he could do about it.

"Let me see," Buckley was saying. "Maybe I can find a way."

Smith knew better than to expect a break, not from this group. Buckley honored that precedent. She folded her hands over her keyboard and fixed her eyes on him before she said,

"There's no provision for misinformation in the system. You'll have to go through regular channels."

Fixated on the smudge of blue icing gracing her cheek, Smith asked what that meant.

"I can set you up with a GP who will get you to a CCS who will refer you in for the ECG stress test."

Although he spoke English, as did Buckley, Smith was at a loss as to what she had just told him.

Sensing her client's confusion, Buckley giggled for a few seconds. Covering her mouth, she discovered the icing on her cheek. She wiped it with her index finger, paused a moment to examine the goop on her finger, then licked it clean.

"What I said was that I'll request an appointment with a General Practitioner who can then point you to a Cardiac Care Specialist who will prescribe the test."

"Thank you," Smith heard himself say. When his brain caught hold of what Buckley said he added, "Timmy's already been to a cardiologist who thinks the test is necessary. Why not just schedule the test?"

"Today is my birthday, Mr. Smith, not yours," Buckley replied with sudden severity. "Would you like me to request a GP appointment or not?"

There was nothing wrong with the system, Smith told himself as he walked down the stairs. It was the people managing it who didn't know what they were doing. If Faber had done his job correctly, then Timmy would have an appointment for his stress test. And if people like Buckley, who had all the information they needed to make an informed decision, would simply proceed to the next logical step, the results would be the same as if they started back at the beginning. But Faber was incompetent and Buckley unwilling, which left Timmy in the lurch.

Walking past the concrete block outside the main entrance, Smith wanted to heave it through the window. It made no sense to commit an act of vandalism to relieve his frustration, but there was something he could do to foil Rieser's corruption. He grabbed the block, carried it across the lot, and deposited it in the back of his truck. When Monday came, Rieser and Plant would have to find another way to conceal their scam. As for the people, they would find themselves in line, first come, first served, the way it was supposed to be. Fair.

Having a few hours to spare, Smith decided to pay a visit to Doctor Ben. If for no other reason, he wanted to see how much progress had been made on the mill. There was also the possibility of having a friendly chat with him, during which Smith would mention Timmy's progress and ask in a friendly way if Doctor Ben might be able to do the favor of getting his son to a cardiologist first instead of second. A favor was all he was looking for, not a quid pro quo the way Ralph would want it, just something one person does for another out of kindness and generosity.

Turning off Route 1 onto the two-lane road that led to the Thorpe Estate, Smith saw the orange cones of a work crew ahead. He rolled to a stop at the request of a flagman and immediately switched off the pickup's engine to save gas. A pair of utility trucks, their booms up in the air, blocked the right lane. Smith watched the men working high above the ground on the power lines. He wasn't afraid of heights, but he preferred to work with his feet in the dirt.

"Hurry up!" the flagman urged.

Smith lowered his eyes, saw the man waving at him, and turned the key. When the engine didn't catch on the first try the flagman dropped his arms.

"Ah, man," he said. "Are we going to have to push you?"

To Smith's relief, the engine caught and he was rolling a few seconds later. Passing the flagman with an apologetic wave, he noticed the decal on the door of one of the utility trucks: CER-TIFIED RURAL BEAUTIFICATION CONTRACTOR.

Doctor Ben was nowhere in sight when Smith parked near the barn. A series of large tents were pitched in the lawn not far from his house. He didn't know what to make of that as he knocked on the door and waited for a reply. After several unsuccessful tries, he poked his head into the barn where he found only a trio of sparrows. He hiked along the path that cut across the property toward the pond, figuring Ben would be there or at the mill itself.

A scene from the nineteenth century greeted him at the pond. On the west side, a pair of stout horses led by a teamster pulled a crude dredge steered by another man who stood deep in the muck of the drained pond. Smith watched as the dredge was hauled to shore, the mud discharged, and then dragged down by a separate team of horses on the east side. Several men shoveled the discharged mud into the back of a wagon.

Doctor Ben stood where the pond emptied into the sluice. He wore a pair of heavy jeans tucked into tall boots, the whole affair held up by a pair of suspenders, the straps of which stretched over his chest. His physique was impressive given his age, and he presided over the work like a general surveying a battlefield in anticipation of the next attack.

"What brings you out here?" Ben asked. "Looking for some exercise?"

"Just wanted to see how things were going," Smith replied.

"That's a long way to go for someone on your gas ration," Ben joked. "Since you made the trek, let me give you the tour."

They followed the same path as during his first visit. Doctor Ben led the way, relying on his cane only a few times when the going was tricky. Smith wished he had a staff of his own if only for balance as he clambered over stray tree roots that mired the path.

While it had been only six weeks, it might have been six months for all the work that had been done to the mill. The building had been reduced to four walls, which were now in perfect condition thanks to some exceptional masonry work. The dilapidated roof, broken wheel, and the rest of the debris now lay in a neat pile at the edge of the road leading back toward the barn. By Smith's count, eight men worked at various tasks. Two used hand drawn planes to shape a massive timber that seemed appropriate for the roof. Three others fit a frame into the doorway, while the same number struggled with a window on the upper floor.

"We're just getting started," Ben said, pointing his cane at the men shaping the roof truss. "More wood is on the way and some iron, too. Then we'll get to building the wheel."

"Amish?" Smith asked.

"That's right," Ben answered. "Not the most precise, mind you, but very capable."

"Sure looks that way."

"The best part is they don't need gasoline or diesel fuel or electricity. I have plenty of acres for grazing and lots of oats for those horses. Plus the manure will be good for my garden."

"Very eco-savvy of you," Smith commented.

Ben leaned on his cane and said, "Doing what makes sense." He crossed to the doorway of the mill, exchanged a few words with the lead man there, and then waved for Smith to follow him toward the house.

"Was that Pennsylvania Dutch you were speaking?" Smith asked as they walked along the dirt road.

"That's right," Ben answered. "Most of the men here speak English, but they're more comfortable with their own tongue."

"Must be rare these days," Smith reflected.

"In another decade or so you won't hear a word of it. Being a doctor to them over the past thirty years, as much as they'll let me, I picked it up."

Three wagons waited beside the barn, each containing lumber destined for the mill. Ben gave them a cursory inspection then waved the drivers on.

"Okay," he said to Smith, "You've had enough time to relax. Let's go inside and you can tell me the real reason you burned two gallons of gas to come out here."

Smith did as he was told, retrieving Timmy's paperwork from his truck before entering the house. Doctor Ben was already seated at the kitchen table where an enormous calico cat sprawled across one end of it. After retrieving an apple from a wooden bowl, he opened a pocketknife and proceeded to slice the fruit into neat sections.

"Take a seat," Ben said. "Don't mind Marvin. He's been fed."

The cat yawned and stretched his forelegs then put his head down. Smith gave him a rub between the ears as Doctor Ben ate his apple.

"Forget the file. Tell me what was said."

"The cardiologist said that Timmy doesn't have a heart valve problem."

"He actually listened to his heart?"

"He did," Smith confirmed.

"Any other tests?"

"That's why I came to see you," Smith admitted.

Ben smiled. "I knew we'd get to it sooner or later. Go ahead."

It took Smith a few seconds to start his explanation. He thought it would be a waste not to use a connection, no matter how tenuous it might be. The problem was making the approach without being a worm.

At last, he said, "The cardiologist thought that Timmy might have a type of arrhythmia. He recommended several tests."

"An electrocardiogram?"

"That combined with a stress test because Timmy collapsed while he was running on the baseball field."

"Sounds like the right thing."

"It does, but Timmy has to go back to a primary care doctor and then another cardiologist before he can get the tests."

Doctor Ben stopped cutting his apple. "That's Universal Coverage for you," he said. "Very thorough."

Hoping for a different answer, Smith glanced at Marvin to avoid Doctor Ben's gaze. "Timmy seems fine," he continued. "He tells me nothing hurts, but I'd like to have those tests done to be sure everything's okay."

"You'll get them," Ben said. "In due time."

All the way to his wellness meeting, Smith sulked for not having the nerve to ask Doctor Ben for help on Timmy's case. In the end he couldn't do it, not because he didn't want to, but because it was the wrong thing to do. It was that, and if he wanted to be completely honest, it was also his pride. Ben sat there, munching his apple, staring at him expectantly, probably knowing that a favor was about to be requested. There was nothing condescending about him. It was simply that Smith felt like a beggar, which in a way he was, in the court of a man in complete control of his small piece of the world. That was what stopped Smith from initiating his request, that feeling of inferiority, of desperation, of having to pester someone for an accommodation to obtain what was supposed to be his right.

Driving to the FART station he recalled the UCM regulation that Hannah had quoted after Doctor Ben's visit to their home. Visiting physicians were not permitted to practice outside their district. Had he asked for a referral, Ben couldn't give it even if he wanted to. This reality salved his ego a bit.

Still, as he rode the train into town, he admitted there was more to it. He'd been on the sidelines at work for a month and a half. While Josh kept Central West on schedule, Smith doodled on a scratch pad. In a matter of days, the President of the United States would be back in town to turn the first shovel of dirt. If Timmy's paperwork wasn't squared away in time, Smith might as well take that day off, too.

He arrived at the former Saint Margaret's church in a cheerless mood, which was appropriate for the subject matter of the wellness meeting, except that it no longer applied to him. Timmy was fine more or less. Fortunately, Leslie sat next to him, bringing a bit of cheer with her.

"This could be my last meeting," she said.

"Mine, too," Smith responded hopefully as the meeting came to order.

"To be free in life is to accept the inevitability of death," Dr. Solorzano intoned using the voice of a chanting monk. "Let us state our acceptance of death."

The group joined hands and replied in unison, "We affirm our lives by accepting death."

Two hours of confessions and affirmations later, Smith

showed his Universal Coverage Card to the receptionist who copied his policy number onto her billing sheet. As he turned to exit the building, Leslie called out to him, asking if he would wait for her.

"Sure," Smith said.

"It's a pleasure to see independent support groups form organically," Dr. Solorzano commented to him. "I think I'll develop take home materials that can be reviewed the following week. Would that be helpful?"

Smith's first reaction was that Dr. Solorzano was a crackpot obsessed with the spectacle of other people's misery, but he wouldn't dare reveal the thought. Instead he regarded Solorzano with a pious gaze and said that the meetings were quite effective as they were.

"I worry we don't do enough," Solorzano replied before excusing himself.

Outside, Leslie guided Smith down the sidewalk to a man who wore a Phillies cap and polo shirt. "This is my husband, Phil," she said.

"Pleased to meet you," Smith said.

"Likewise," Phil returned. "What do you say we grab a drink and talk about healthcare?" When Smith hesitated, he added, "This won't be like one of those meetings you have to sit through."

Smith wasn't afraid of more talk about death. Rather, he believed a person's healthcare was a private matter. On top of that, he didn't want to miss the next train west, or he would be stuck in town another hour and a half.

"When was the last time you had a drink out?" Phil prodded. "I'll buy."

It would be rude not to accept the man's offer and the FART

was frequently late. "One and then I have to catch the train."

"Perfect."

They stepped into the Stars and Stripes, a mock eighteenth century tavern that served draft beer in ceramic mugs under faux paintings of Revolutionary War scenes.

"Leslie let slip that I went to the *Salvare* for treatment," Phil said after tasting his beer.

Leslie gave her husband a sheepish look then stared at the floor between her feet.

"Don't worry, babe," Phil said. "You and I grew up when you could say whatever you wanted in this country." Turning his head to face Smith again, he asked, "Did you happen to tell anyone about that?"

"No," Smith answered truthfully. He'd more or less forgotten this small fact, and now didn't see the relevance of it.

"Thanks for that," Phil said. "I'd appreciate it if you would forget that my dear couldn't hold her tongue."

Leslie said, "I was excited that you were going to be okay, and I was stuck in that awful meeting, saying stupid things over and over. It was nice to talk to someone halfway normal for a change."

"Relax. It's alright. He was stuck there with you, and he's a decent guy. He understands. Don't you, Bob?"

Smith recalled that a visit to the *Salvare* might lead to trouble with the Universal Coverage System. It was part of the disclosure portion of Dr. Jossy's commercials. While he thought someone taking a chance on the *Salvare* didn't necessarily deserve punishment, he wasn't about to aid them in escaping the law.

"Why would anyone ask me about you?" he inquired.

"The Healthcare Administration Authority has a division called the Medical Service Bureau. They have an investigation underway. They're questioning everyone who ever knew Leslie and me. The only thing they care about is issuing fines. It makes them look good."

Thinking that there was more to Phil's story than a mere visit to the *Salvare* for treatment, Smith said, "I don't want anything to do with your treatment outside the system or anything else you're involved in."

Phil kept Smith in his seat with a firm hand on his shoulder. "All I did was get help when I needed it most, which was right away, not sometime later, probably when it would have been too late. You can't blame me for that. If anything, this was about survival."

"Then you have nothing to worry about," Smith said.

"Except those MSB guys asking questions about how I was so quickly and miraculously cured without having been treated in the Universal Coverage System," Phil countered. "If they find out I was aboard the *Salvare* without approval they'll punish me for saving my own life instead of waiting for the nails in my coffin the way Dr. Solorzano back there wants us all to do."

"He just wants to help people cope."

Phil snorted. "No one here believes that including you. He gets two hundred dollars a head for everyone at the meeting. Not a bad racket for a guy with a dime store diploma and a leaking roof."

Smith shifted in his seat. "I don't know his credentials or if his roof leaks."

"It doesn't matter. All I'm asking you, man to man, is that you develop a mild case of amnesia should someone from the MSB come calling. You don't have to lie. Just tell them you don't remember anything about old Phil except that you shared some meetings with his lovely wife."

One thing nagged Smith about Phil's claim and he decided to ask about it. "If all you need is an approval to avoid the fine, why didn't you get one?"

Phil shook his head the way Coach Dolante did when a new kid whiffed through an easy pitch. "Waiting for someone to push the papers around didn't seem like a good idea," he answered, "when the cancer might have killed me in the meantime. Besides, I hear the way the game works is you don't get approval. That way they can write you a fine when you do what you have to do."

He'd heard enough and Smith pushed back from the table. "Thanks for the beer," he said.

"One last thing, Bob. Between you and me, that ship is the best thing going for anyone who needs real healthcare, the kind we had before this Universal Coverage thing got started. They have everything you need out there and more. The doctors speak English, the nurses care about you, and the place is spotless. You should see the fancy equipment. It will blow your mind."

"I'm sure it would," Smith said, adding with a twist of his mouth. "Cheap, too, right?"

"Fair enough when you consider the alternative."

CHAPTER
FOURTEEN

SMITH WIDENED THE MOUTH OF THE TRASH BAG he held. His son deposited several bottles and a bunch of candy wrappers into it then kicked a nearby can several yards ahead of them.

"Timmy! Go get that can. Right now."

"Why do we have to pick up other people's trash?" Timmy moaned.

"Get that can," Smith ordered his son. When it was in the bag, he said, "We're here to do our part to make our community a better place."

"But we don't live around here."

"We live nearby," Smith reminded his boy while simultaneously weighing the idea of telling him that they may be moving to the city soon. He made a lesson of the subject. "What if we lived here?"

"I don't want to live here," Timmy answered.

"That's not the question."

The last time he performed his monthly community service, Timmy had fun. He and some high school guys painted an old lady's house. They used words he knew he wasn't supposed to say, not even when he missed an easy pitch or bobbled a pop-up fly ball. The first time he repeated one of them, they laughed and asked him if he knew what it meant. When he shrugged that he didn't, they told him then laughed at his reaction. Timmy chuckled, too, even though he didn't fully understand the definition. They promptly told him to keep it to himself, and no matter what, never use the term around women. He'd looked over his shoulder to see if his mom had seen him. He spotted her through a back window in the house. She was outside, chatting with several other adults.

"Answer me, Timmy," his father was saying, "What if we lived here?"

"I know dad. I'd like it to be nice and stuff the way it is by our house." This was the answer he knew his father wanted to hear, but it made no sense to clean up someone else's street. He didn't hit home runs for the other team, did he? Along those lines, he would rather be in the batting cage, practicing his swing so he'd be ready for the next game.

For his part, Smith had other things on his mind as well. The first shovel ceremony was less than a week away, and Henny Geerman had yet to receive notice that Timmy was off the life-threatening condition list. She promised to check on it first thing Monday morning. If she was unable to make any progress, Smith planned on speaking directly with Mr. Wexler.

"How much farther do we have to go?" Timmy asked.

"Eight more blocks," Smith replied.

"We're gonna need some more bags, dad."

Father and son arrived home just past six. It was Hannah's turn for a night out and she busiest herself getting ready. Although Smith rarely availed himself of the same opportunity, he didn't mind his wife going out with her friends. It went a long way toward domestic harmony, and he preferred to spend weekend evenings with Timmy or in his home office catching up on the latest developments in engineering.

Hannah departed just as Smith and Timmy settled in on the couch to watch the Phillies play the Orioles. To make it like a night at the ballpark, they made hotdogs and popcorn and had a large bag of roasted peanuts sitting between them. The windows were open, letting a warm breeze flow through the room, which, with the TV volume all the way up, made the experience as real as it could be without taking Ralph's offer of tickets near the dugout.

The second inning had just begun when Hannah suddenly returned. Stomping into the room she snatched the remote control away from Timmy, pointed it at the TV, and silenced the action.

"Awww, mom, Terry Bucci is at bat!" Timmy protested.

"What's wrong?" Smith asked his wife.

Hannah dropped the remote. In its place she held up her M Fuel Card. "This doesn't work anymore."

"Doesn't work?"

"Is there an echo in here?" Hannah mocked him. "I barely made it home from the fuel depot where I couldn't get gas. How am I going to get out with my girlfriends tonight?"

"Take the FART," Smith said. "It's been on time lately."

"On time?" Hannah puffed, pointing to her watch. "I'm going to be late no matter what, and it's my turn to drive."

"I thought you were meeting in the city."

"We are, and I was going to give everyone a ride to a new place in Devon."

"You're driving into town then all the way back out to Devon?"

"If we lived in the city, I wouldn't have this problem."

"Honey, the extra gas is supposed to be used for medical reasons, not for a night out on the town."

"If the card isn't working, which it's not, how can I get gas for anything?"

"Ask your girlfriends to help out with one of their vouchers," Smith suggested.

"Are you kidding me?"

"Look, I'll drop you off at the FART station, you can meet them in town and try another place."

Timmy watched his mother stare at his father the way Detective Elroy had at that guy who stole the old man's baseball cards. The argument they were having bothered him less than the fact that she was going out for the evening instead of staying in with them. Another cheering voice in the room would only add to the fun, especially because they were all Phillies fans. However, baseball ranked low on his mom's priorities. He caught her gabbing with her friends when he was at bat or stretching his lead from third base toward home plate. But she was a girl and how could he expect her to be into the game as much as he was?

"Give me the keys to your truck," Hannah said with her hand out.

"There's only enough room for three people."

"Damn it!"

"Take it easy, honey," Smith said, rising off the couch. "I have an idea."

"Oh, the great engineer Bob Smith has found a way to turn water into gasoline."

If Timmy hadn't been there, Smith would have cursed the way his father did when he smashed his knuckles under the hood of someone's car. With Timmy there, and paying attention despite the fact that Terry Bucci had two strikes, he kept his language clean.

"Come on," he said and headed for the garage.

He stepped around his pickup, shifted several toolboxes, and retrieved one of the five gallon jugs he'd filled during the previous month. Right behind him, Hannah spotted the second one, which Smith had also kept out of sight from anyone who might enter the garage unannounced. After all, it was illegal to hoard liquid fuels.

"Your secret stash?" Hannah asked.

"I've ridden the FART for a month straight to save this much gas," Smith retorted. Actually, he'd siphoned the gas out of her SUV, but he also conserved an equal amount, which now sat in his pickup's tank.

"And never told your wife."

"I was saving it for an emergency, in case Timmy needs to go to the hospital or to Pittsburgh again. By the way, you never told me that was a group appointment out there."

Hannah said, "Now you're going to redesign the healthcare system? Timmy is okay, isn't he?"

"We won't know for sure until he gets the ECG," answered Smith. "Did that doctor in Pittsburgh actually listen to his heart?"

"Next you'll be asking me if he spoke English, which didn't matter because there was an interpreter. Could you hurry up?"

Putting the empty jug down, Smith said, "That should be enough." It wasn't lost on him that she hadn't answered his question, which was the same one Doctor Ben had asked.

"Five gallons?"

"Are you planning on driving more than a hundred miles?"

"Are you planning on coming to get me if I run out?"

Without another word, Smith fetched the second jug.

Having heard his name, Timmy left the couch for a better angle on the garage. He originally thought they were arguing about the gas, but then Pittsburgh was mentioned, and he knew he was involved. His mom's voice carried through the open window, delivering the news that he was okay. At the same time, his dad was talking about some kind of test. He wanted to avoid any more tests like Mrs. Marselek's red pen on his homework. Seeing his dad exit the garage, Timmy bolted for the couch.

"What did I miss?" Smith asked Timmy, struggling to forget about his row with Hannah.

"Uh ... nothing much. Seven innings to go, dad."

Although upset with Hannah, Smith felt a small measure of happiness. If her fuel card no longer worked that meant Timmy's name was off the endangered list, and he had every reason to expect he would be reinstalled as foundation team leader on Monday morning.

"Go Phillies!" he shouted.

"Yeah!" Timmy chimed in.

The Phillies won in a game that wasn't decided until the last inning. The thrill of victory did little to relieve either Timmy's or Smith's bellyaches. Between the two of them, they managed to eat all the hotdogs and most of the popcorn and peanuts.

"I'm going to bed," Timmy said, dragging himself off the couch when the post-game show ended.

"See you in the morning champ," Smith said. "Don't forget we're going to clean the cars in the morning."

"I know, dad."

A little queasy himself, Smith took his time returning the living room to some semblance of order. He paid little attention to the TV until his eye caught the tall, white bow of the *Salvare* cutting through a calm sea.

"*Salvare*," the narrator said. "The care you deserve at a price you can afford."

Smith put down the empty popcorn bowl and stared at the screen.

"*Salvare* offers you the most comfortable environment to receive chemotherapy and radiation treatments. Our facilities welcome you not only for the care you need, but for a pleasant recovery stay. Why not make your medical regimen as pleasant as can be? Forget those barracks-like conditions of your present facility and escape to the privacy of your own cabin where you can take in a restorative sea breeze. Bring your spouse or a friend who can stay at no additional charge."

The commercial reminded Smith of Leslie's husband. If the ad was to be believed, Phil had been out there cruising the Atlantic, receiving great care while his wife was holding hands and chanting like a bunch of teenagers at a séance. Smith wondered why Leslie hadn't availed herself of the free stay. Then he remembered that attendance at Dr. Solorzano's wellness meetings affected an employer's Health Policy Rating. Leslie couldn't join her husband if she wanted to.

As the government-required disclaimer began, Smith tapped

the remote. The screen went dark and he headed for the bedroom.

"Check this out," Ralph said as Smith joined him at the coffee pot. "I have two seats for the Eagles pre-season game against Washington."

"Timmy's a Phillies fan," Smith reminded his coworker.

"I have nothing left in the baseball department. Is your boy a hundred percent or do you want my lady friend to see what she can do for him?"

"He was just cleared by the cardiologist last week."

"Great!" Ralph slapped his boss on the back then added, "Don't forget, if you need anything from Universal Coverage, you know, maybe for yourself or Hannah, don't hesitate to ask. Thanks to my procurement abilities, my lady's bosses will be at the Super Bowl."

"You don't even know who will be playing."

"Seats are seats, and yours truly has delivered to the powers that be and they're in the mood to be grateful, if you know what I mean."

"Maybe she can help us with the department fitness level."

"Talk to Lynn about that," Ralph whined. "I'm down two pounds ... uh ... hello, Mr. Wexler."

Smith turned to see Mark Wexler standing at the stairwell door.

"Come straight up to my office, Bob," he said.

"On my way," Smith replied, figuring he was going to be reinstated as team leader by the boss himself.

"We have a problem," Wexler began without offering his former foundation team leader a seat.

Smith replied instinctively. "What can I do to help?" he asked.

"The first shovel won't be turned on Thursday," Wexler continued.

"Why not?"

"That's the problem. The loyal opposition, as they call themselves in Congress, has managed to get an Auditor General to stick his nose into some projects. They're going after Central West with a vengeance."

The estimates and budgets produced by his team were Smith's first concern. He'd reviewed them himself and had asked Josh to do the same. He was confident his team had nothing to worry about. At the same time, he wasn't standing in this particular office because all was well.

"Everything is open to criticism," Wexler was saying. "Everything."

"Give me a chance to check that report," he said.

"Your team's work is fine," Wexler said waving his hand. "The trouble is your son's medical condition."

Caught off guard, Smith grunted and said, "What does that have to do with an audit?"

"That's what I'm trying to understand. Henny has the details, and I'll let her fill you in. The point is, you better get it straightened out immediately."

"I'll do everything I can," Smith assured him.

"Good, because I don't want a single black mark against this firm. Understand? I shoveled a mile of manure for this governor and Wexler Associates won the design against all comers. I'm going to see it built our way."

"Let me tell you, Mr. Wexler, that Timmy has just been cleared by his doctor. I'm ready to get back on the project and see it through."

"Talk to Henny before making me any promises," Wexler said, dismissing Smith with a nod toward the door.

All the way to Geerman's office, Smith searched for something he could have done wrong in the course of Timmy's treatment. He'd followed every rule to the letter. All appointments had been scheduled through the HAO, and he'd kept them accordingly.

Confused, he took his regular seat before Geerman's desk. She'd been waiting for him as was indicated by his open file on her blotter.

"Here's the thing," she said. "You were on a CGP when Timmy first took ill."

"That's right. So what?"

"Your appointment in Pittsburgh was scheduled according to your status. Your furlough from that status should have been made known to the Care Administration Specialist."

"She had me listed as a CGP employee," Smith argued.

"Because I listed you as one here at the firm, Bob, when you were assigned to Central West. But it's your responsibility under Section 1412 of the Universal Coverage Manual to make the CAS aware of any change in your status whenever you meet with them."

"I didn't know that, and the lady didn't ask me either."

"Review section 1412, the section called RESPONSIBILITIES OF THE CLIENT."

Smith never considered Timmy a client of any system. He was a boy, a person, a patient perhaps, but not a client. Lawyers had clients; doctors had patients. Didn't they?

"What's the big deal anyway? Timmy is better now, aside of a few tests. By autumn this will all be in the past."

"Hardly," Geerman said, turning a page in his file. "It'll be everything I can do to keep the firm out of trouble with the Medical Service Bureau."

"I still don't understand what I did wrong."

Geerman turned her monitor to face Smith and ticked off his offenses with her pen. "By not clarifying your employment status, you were granted priority status, Bob. Then your wife applied for an M Fuel Supplement Card in your name, which was expedited for the same reason. Those things normally take a couple of months to be authorized. Then Timmy's cardiac review came through on an accelerated basis. These are stacked violations of the protocol."

"What are we, in the military now?" protested Smith.

"No, but we have rules to follow," Geerman snapped then corrected herself quietly with, "Laws, actually."

Surrendering to the concept without admitting to guilt, he said, "Now what?"

"You have a Health Administration Disciplinary Board hearing tomorrow afternoon."

Unable to resist the jibe, Smith muttered, "They can certainly schedule a hearing faster than an ECG appointment."

"Watch what you say, Bob. I'm emailing your Employee Attitude Analysis to the board today."

"My what?"

"Look, the board is going to ask you some questions about what happened. Tell them the truth. All of it."

"Why would I lie?"

"I'm not saying you would. Just tell them how things unfolded here. Mr. Wexler gave you a temporary furlough, but you were still available for consultation. The best we can hope for is that they put it down to an honest mistake ..."

"Which it was," Smith interrupted.

"... and they'll give us a warning as opposed to a fine or a negative rating of our Health Policy Implementation Practices, in which case every Wexler employee will be assigned an additional premium based upon the board's determination of intent."

It was hard to believe that one boy seeing a couple of doctors could have precipitated such a reaction, but April Fools Day was months ago, and Henny was not known for her jokes. Confirmation came when her printer spit out a Medical Service Bureau Summons, which she positioned at the edge of her desk.

"How could they possibly accuse the firm of intentionally doing something wrong?" Smith dared to ask.

"I've heard these people are worse than the IRS, Bob."

"Does that mean I need a lawyer?"

Geerman didn't think a lawyer was a good idea. "Having an attorney will make you look guilty," she said.

Upon hearing this, Smith let out a rolling belly laugh that brought tears to his eyes. The combination of her sternness and the ridiculous nature of the situation were too absurd to take seriously. The fun ended when the human resources director hit him with the next blow.

"Timmy has to be there, too. Technically, he's responsible for the violations."

Smith sucked a deep breath, looked hard at his HR director, and said, "Timmy is eleven years old, Mrs. Geerman. He's responsible for getting A's on his report card, cleaning his room, and staying out of trouble. His team counts on him for a few home runs and a good arm when he's on the field. Other than that, he's a kid, and this kangaroo court or whatever I have to deal with tomorrow had better understand that."

On that note, he snatched his summons off her desk and left without another word. He charged up the stairs, where anyone who saw him coming was smart enough to stay out of the way.

"THAT GUY WAS A JERK."

CHAPTER
FIFTEEN

AT HOME THAT EVENING, Smith dug out the Universal Coverage Manual. He sat with his feet up on his desk, the manual on his lap, and a cold glass of iced-tea sweating in his left hand. Emboldened by his earlier audacity, he read through Section 1412 with a critical eye. There was no doubt that the regulations had been breached. He should have informed the HAO of his change in status, turned in the M Fuel Card, and accepted his fate. The real question, and the one he intended to put to the board, was who bore responsibility for the error. Yes, he had not reported his change in status, but nor had Henny Geerman, and neither Ms. Buckley nor Ms. Ledsoe had asked about it. While none of the aforementioned people were specifically required to do so, a case could be made that they had been partially responsible for what occurred, and should have to accept some of the fault. No matter what, Timmy was blameless.

Smith specifically remembered when the President signed the Universal Coverage Act. He and Hannah joined tens of thousands of others crowded into the National Mall for a first hand view of the ceremony, which was held on the steps of the Capitol building. Thankfully, huge television screens provided up-close live coverage. After signing the bill into law the President said that, "every person is now guaranteed the best possible care." For those who had forgotten, his speech was reprinted on the first page of the UCM. If he was guilty of anything, Smith thought, it was pursuit of that goal, doing the best he could for Timmy, which was his job as a father.

Smith enjoyed being Timmy's dad. His son gave him every reason to be proud and hopeful. It was more than his success in school or on the baseball field. It was the vague idea that there was a future beyond Smith's own mortality, a legacy of sorts that didn't have to be as grandiose as much as it had to be authentic. Smith knew that his son was not a copy of himself but certainly an impression of him the way Smith was of his own father. Soon enough, Timmy would be his own man, doing what it was he found to be important in the world. He couldn't expect the boy to figure that out yet. However, he did expect Timmy to live to be an old man who looked back on his own children and accomplishments with an equally sentimental eye.

At the sound of Timmy and Hannah entering the house, Smith tossed the UCM on his desk. What did he want with a thousand pages of regulations when he could practice baseball with his only son?

On his way into Health Administration District Office 117, Smith noticed that the cement block he'd taken had been re- placed with a plain piece of stone. He didn't dare look beneath it. There were too many people waiting on the sidewalk and Timmy was at his side. They entered the building and once again came upon Mr. Fetterman.

"I know you," Fetterman joked. "You're the best hitter the Media Moguls has."

Beaming, Timmy replied, "Thanks, Mr. Fetterman."

"If I had a baseball, I'd ask you to sign it for me."

On any other occasion, Timmy would have a ball with him, his glove, too, but he had to go to this stupid hearing with his dad. Thus, his equipment was at home, except for his lucky fifty- cent piece that he always stuck in the pocket of his jeans.

"Sorry, I don't have one," he said.

"That's okay. Let me shake your hand.

As the two shook hands, Smith asked, "Are you going to the game tonight?"

"If my legs will take me there."

"Maybe I could give you a ride."

Fetterman refused the offer. "I'm in training," he said, add- ing with his chin pointed at Timmy, "Good luck tonight against the Titans."

"We're gonna win," Timmy grinned. Being recognized off the field put him in the big leagues, up there with the professional sluggers. It wasn't only Coach Dolante telling him he was a cham- pion anymore. He had fans.

"Don't let it go to your head," his dad said as he steered him toward their door.

Their next stop was Rieser's desk, where the hearing sum- mons was accepted with a sneer.

"One of the lucky ones," Rieser said. "Down the hall, first door to the right, take a seat and wait for your name to be called."

Smith figured luck would have nothing to do with the verdict. More likely it would come down to personality, in particular his and how it meshed with the members of the board. Sitting on a plastic chair in the hallway outside the hearing room, he thought back to his days working at his father's service station. Conjuring up the charm he'd used then was easy. He had fond memories of his weekends and summers there. Just as he formed a mental picture of the Penner sisters pulling up in their matching Camaros, the hearing room door opened and a security guard who could have been Rieser's twin called his son's name.

"Smith, Timothy."

"That's me," Timmy said getting up, thinking this guy would soon know him by sight, too, like all the great players.

"Who are you?" the cop asked Smith from behind a pointed finger.

"I'm his father."

"Oh, you're an 816 in a 1412 case. Let's go."

Smith and Timmy followed the guard into an auditorium that could have swallowed the one at Timmy's school in a single gulp. They hurried down the long aisle, trying to keep up with the guard who told them to take a seat in the first row while he climbed the stairs at the side of the stage.

Four people sat behind a simple table positioned in the middle of the stage. Smith assumed the one all the way to his left was the official record keeper because he had a laptop computer open in front of him and a small printer off to the side. He accepted Smith's summons from the guard and tapped at his keyboard before passing it along to the other three. Each of them looked it over for a few seconds.

No one wore robes, which put Smith at ease. They all looked liked him, regular people doing a job. They probably didn't want to be here anymore than he did.

"I'm Executive Inspector Greg Besset from the Medical Service Bureau, assigned to Health Administration District Office 117," said the man in the center of the table. "These proceedings are authorized under the Universal Healthcare and Medical Assistance Act, specifically to monitor and improve …"

The other members rolled their eyes, yawned, or chewed pens. Undeterred by these reactions Besset completed his introduction then read from a single sheet of paper given to him by the clerk.

"Let the record show that this disciplinary hearing has been called due to violations which can be found under Section 1412 of the UC Code, et cetera."

"Duly noted," the clerk intoned.

"We have a Universal Coverage client, Timothy Smith, who requested an appointment with a cardiac specialist under the auspices of his father … I assume that's you?"

Smith replied, "I'm Timothy's father."

Besset picked up with, "That his father was currently in the employ of a CGP as defined under Section 508."

"What's a CGP?" Timmy whispered to his dad.

"Just sit quiet for now, okay?"

"As it turns out, the father of the aforementioned client, who comes under Section 816 and is responsible for the client's actions within the system, did not have this status at the time of the scheduling event."

Smith rose and said, "If I can clarify …"

"Please remain seated, Mr. Smith," Besset said.

"Sorry."

"There are several other violations, all of which fall back to Section 1412. We have an illegally obtained M Fuel Supplement Card, a subsequent cardiac review, so on and so on. Let's deal with this 1412 thing. Are we in agreement?"

The others nodded that they were.

"Good," Besset said then returned his focus to Smith. "Now it's your turn. Tell us how you ended up here and keep it short."

Smith stood up and moved a few steps forward. "I work for Wexler Associates, the engineering firm that won the contract for the Central West project in Philadelphia."

"Oh, that's all we needed to know," mocked Besset. "By the way, they are Urban Redevelopment and Enhancement Areas, not projects."

Plodding on, Smith said, "You all should know that Central West has been deemed a CGP, part of the recent stimulus act. You might remember the President was here a few months ago for the announcement of the funding."

Besset rediscovered his official countenance and put it back on display. "Go on," he said.

"I'm the team leader of the foundation department," Smith explained. "My son, Timmy, collapsed on the baseball field the same day the President met with many of us at the Wexler Building. After a visit to the emergency room, I followed the doctor's recommendations and scheduled his next appointment."

"Hold on," interrupted Besset. "Dr. Zulfikar's notes in the file state that the client was to follow up with his general practitioner in ninety days, but you requested an initial cardiac analysis."

"I came to this building and asked the person for a heart specialist to get a second opinion."

"Let the record stress that the 816 client representative acknowledges committing the precipitating act."

"Wait a minute," Smith put in. "All I did was follow the system to get my son a doctor."

"You didn't follow the system, Mr. Smith. That's why you're here. Had you come to this building, visited with an Administration Care Specialist and scheduled an initial evaluation with a general practitioner for your son, then you could stand here and tell us that you followed the system. Of course, you would have clarified your CGP status under Section 508 at the time it changed. Had you done all these things as described you wouldn't be here in the first place."

"At the time I scheduled the appointment I was on the CGP. I am still available for consultation."

Besset was unimpressed. "Your employment status changed before the client was present for his cardiac review. Your employer amended your Citizen Health Profile properly. It is your obligation under section 1412 to notify the Health Administration District Office, specifically the Care Administration Specialist, of your change in status immediately."

"Then Timmy would not have seen the doctor until ..."

Shaking his head, Besset rejected Smith's claim, "Not only would Timmy have seen a doctor, he would have seen the correct doctor had you properly followed the system. For your sake, I'll review what you should have done: 1) The client sees his GP; 2) The GP recommends any follow up care; 3) Follow up care is scheduled through the HAO; and 4) All of the above is conducted under one's PROPER employment status or any other factors that are to be correctly and accurately stated to the CAS. Have I made this clear enough for you?"

Smith realized he'd been holding his breath so as to not say something stupid. He blew out the stale air and took a fresh lungful before he said, "What if Timmy needed immediate surgery? How would that work?"

"You want to talk about hypothetical situations?" questioned Besset. "We don't have time for that."

Considering no one else was in the room, Smith thought there was plenty of time to discuss all sorts of possibilities, but he knew better than to express that sentiment.

"The point is, Mr. Smith, you violated the law by not notifying the CAS of your change in status. It's that simple and there's nothing hypothetical about it."

"Shouldn't Ms. Buckley or Ms. Ledsoe have asked?" Smith ventured. "Shouldn't the computers have shared that information the way they do everything else?"

"Do I have to read section 1412 to you, Mr. Smith? You seem like a smart guy, you claim to be a team leader of foundations or something for a big construction outfit. You should be able to grasp what the problem is, right?"

"I understand."

"Good. The only thing left is how we're going to process the violation. Give me a minute to check the manual."

The clerk stopped typing, leaned over, and said something to Besset.

"Yes, thanks. I almost forgot about the fuel card."

Besset reminded Smith of Mr. Kuhn who had been one of his father's most persnickety customers. He would make a fuss if a single drop of gas spilled on his car's paint. The other members of the board were a dour pair who showed as much empathy as a couple of jailers.

Looking over his shoulder at Timmy, Smith saw that his son didn't know what to make of the proceedings. He gave him a thumbs-up but Timmy didn't react.

"Up here, Mr. Smith," Besset called, then continued after

a few beats. "The guidance I've found in the manual authorizes several remedies. That being the case, I'm going to mix and match so nothing falls through the cracks."

Figuring this was his last chance, Smith took another step forward in anticipation of the opportunity to speak.

"You'd like to say something?" asked Besset.

"Only that I didn't know I was breaking any rules. I thought I was following the rules. I only wanted to do the right thing for my son."

"Understood. Understood."

That Besset paused to contemplate for a few moments gave Smith comfort that this silly affair might end with a lecture, the kind that would be more appropriate if Timmy acted up in class than one for a grown man who made a few honest mistakes.

"Okay. In the first place, your employer, Wexler Associates, amended the Citizen Health Profile correctly. Thus, there's nothing to be done in regard to them. Let the record reflect that and will the clerk please send notice to them that their involvement in the case is finished."

"Duly noted."

"As for Mr. Robert Smith, an 816 designated caregiver, he shall pay a five hundred dollar fine and as restitution for an illegally authorized M Fuel Card, have his monthly fuel ration docked accordingly."

"That would be 30 gallons drawn under the card," the clerk remarked.

"30 gallons, so be it," Besset repeated to the clerk. "Timothy Smith, a minor under the supervision of Mr. Robert Smith as provided by 816, has no culpability." Then looking at Smith, Besset said, "Take this as a warning. The system is easy. There are people to guide you along the way. Listen to them. Do what they tell you to do. That way, you'll stay out of trouble."

He might have had a stroke for the way Smith stood with unfocused eyes and his mouth open. Or, he might have been struck by lightning. Either way, he found it incredible that for the sake of a few first-time blunders his pickup would be parked for six weeks. Getting to Timmy's games was going to be a real challenge. And the five hundred dollars? Where was that going to come from?

Now angry, but still under control, Smith said, "What about an appeal?"

"An appeal opens you to the possibility of a reconsidered verdict and subsequent increase in the assessed penalties. I don't think you want to risk that, do you?"

Another roll of the dice did not sound enticing. There was the whir of the clerk's printer and from it came several sheets of paper. The guard carried them down the stairs, placed them at the foot of the stage, and drew a pen from his shirt pocket.

"Sign here," he said.

"I'd like to read it first," Smith replied. He took his time, too. Having learned not to skip anything, he used his finger to underline every word. The text was typical legal boilerplate, all of which could be summed up in the space of a parking ticket. He signed his name, accepted his copy, and left the room with Timmy a step behind.

"That guy was a jerk," Timmy said as they exited the building.

CHAPTER SIXTEEN

TIMMY HADN'T THOUGHT MUCH OF THE HEARING until after supper. To that point, it was kind of like being in school. That guy used the same tone of voice as Mrs. Marselek did when she had to interrupt her lesson to stop Kate Ammon from chatting with Heidi Cosgrove. He understood that his dad had done something wrong, and that whatever it was it had to do with his doctor visits. Five hundred dollars was serious money, Timmy knew, because Detective Elroy had held up one of the recovered baseball cards and said it was worth that much. His dad had to pay the money to make up for what he'd done, which was unclear to Timmy since his dad was no criminal like the guy who stole the cards. His mom asked how the hearing went and his dad said they'd talk about it later.

Therefore, it wasn't until his mom and dad left the kitchen together that Timmy realized how much he had been part of the problem. They retreated to his dad's office in the far corner of the first floor and closed the door. He eavesdropped from his bedroom, directly above them.

"If you hadn't panicked, this could have been avoided," his mother was saying.

"I didn't panic."

"You had to get to the HAO right away, didn't you?"

"What if I'd waited and Timmy had another episode."

"He didn't and the reason is because there's nothing wrong with him."

"The emergency room doctor said there was, a leaking heart valve if you remember. I did what I did because of what he said."

"He made a mistake, Bob. Everybody makes mistakes."

"Except that I'm not allowed one now and then."

"If you had followed the ER doctor's instructions and taken Timmy to a GP, his mistake would have been discovered and you wouldn't have been able to make yours."

"If I recall correctly, you wouldn't so much as let Doctor Ben listen to Timmy's heart."

"You'd rather trust some old man riding around with a bag full of bottles than a certified ..."

"He is a licensed doctor, Hannah, a visiting physician in the next district."

"Yeah, and he's not supposed to be over here freelancing or whatever else he had in mind. You're lucky the board didn't find out about that. You'd have another fine to deal with."

"He was doing me a favor, honey."

"He was breaking the law."

"Then it's a stupid law. At least you know the family budget is going to be a little tight for a month or so. I'm taking Timmy to his game."

Upon hearing this, Timmy scrambled to don his uniform. He was supposed to be ready by now, waiting for his dad by the pickup.

"Ready to go, Timmy?" his father called up the stairs.

"I'll be right down!"

The Media Moguls faced the Springfield Titans that evening. A lively crowd of parents filled the bleachers, supplemented by two busloads of younger kids who would be playing at this level next year. Handmade signs bobbed in various quarters, usually in the vicinity of a particularly vocal group. It was all in good fun as this was the best and cheapest form of entertainment in the suburbs.

Mr. Fetterman stood in his usual spot at the fence behind first base. He never missed a Moguls game even though the walk to the field took him nearly an hour. It wasn't very far, just a challenge for a man on eighty-year-old legs. He played the sport in high school and still enjoyed watching it, especially in this purest form. These were kids, each trying to be the best, putting their hearts into it not for a million dollar contract, but for love of the game and the cheers from the stands.

Fetterman watched Timmy step up to the plate. He was the Moguls' best hitter. In the field, Joey Anzalone had a glove that always seemed to find the ball, but he was long gone. The kid who took his place, Les Sobel, did well enough but lacked Anzalone's speed. The Moguls needed Timmy more than ever, both his bat and his talent at shortstop, to keep any challenger in check.

The first two pitches were balls that Timmy let whiz by without a twitch. Then a strike came, dead center over the plate, one that, had the bat been swung, would have been knocked over the wall, something Timmy had shown himself capable of doing on many occasions. For some reason he let it go. Fetterman wondered if his favorite player wasn't trying to lure the pitcher into a trap. There was more strategy to the game than the average fan understood. At any rate, he hoped to see a few homers because this game might be the last one he watched from the outfield wall.

The trouble was that Timmy's stomach did a few flips right after he stepped up to the plate. He thought he might have eaten too much for supper, but then his gut settled and he took a deep breath, which left him feeling better. That was when the second ball slapped the catcher's glove. As the pitcher wound up for the next throw, his vision blurred, enough that he heard the ball come in but couldn't make it out. The umpire called the strike and all Timmy could think about was how dry his mouth had become. He drew a couple more breaths, stepped out of the batter's box for a swing, and everything went back to normal. He had no reason to be nervous. He knew this pitcher; he hit a double off him during their last meeting.

Another strike flew across the plate. For whatever reason, Timmy lacked his usual concentration. A flutter spread out from his chest, bringing with it the stomach flips that bothered him a few minutes ago. He swallowed hard, shook his head, and looked out at the pitcher. It occurred to him that he should tell his dad he didn't feel well the way Dr. Hillman made him promise he would. But after that hearing and the argument his parents had about it, Timmy didn't want to stir up more trouble.

He knew there was nothing really wrong with him. He drank too much water in the dugout, or maybe he was trying too hard to keep the Moguls on top after Joey's departure.

His swing at the next pitch produced a groan from the crowd. This third strike relieved the pressure on him, and he carried his bat to the dugout without looking into the stands for his dad's reaction.

"Sorry, coach," he said taking a seat in line among the other kids on the bench.

"That's okay, Timmy. Next time you'll hit a homer," Coach Dolante told him then pointed at the next batter. "Jeff, let's go. Troy, you're on deck."

From his spot in the right field bleachers, Smith applauded Timmy's effort. He couldn't expect his son to hit home runs every time he came to the plate, but he did feel Timmy's disappointment. Even from that distance he could see the consternation on his son's face. At the same time, striking out was a good lesson, a reminder that there was always someone out there to challenge you. It never hurt to introduce some humility every once in a while, and striking out did that to great effect. Not that Timmy had shown any arrogance on or off the field. Like Smith himself, he was a team player.

As the next boy dug his feet into the dirt beside home plate, Smith noticed a vehicle moving in the parking lot beyond the backstop. It was the ambulance that was always present at the games in case a player was injured. The lights weren't flashing, which confirmed there was no emergency. The driver tapped the siren for a single blast, received a wave in reply from someone standing there, and wheeled toward the road.

A loud crack resonated across the field as Jeff connected with a pitch. The people from Media were on their feet, everyone but Smith. He couldn't understand why the ambulance was leaving in the middle of the fifth inning. It was supposed to be there for the entire game. For Timmy's sake, he would be sure to speak with the crew before the next game.

•◆• •◆• •◆•

Although he had a full tank in the pickup, Smith rode the FART into Philadelphia the next morning. There would be no fuel vouchers in his mailbox for the next six weeks and he wanted to conserve every drop of gas he could to have enough to get to Timmy's games, and God forbid, to take him to the hospital.

Arriving at the coffee pot on the eighth floor of the Wexler Building, he was not surprised to find Ralph holding court with several other guys.

"The Eagles are looking good at training camp," Ralph said.

Playing along, Smith replied, "I couldn't imagine who might have tickets to the first game."

With a bow and a grand smile, Ralph said in his best master of ceremonies voice, "Yours truly!"

"Mind if I get a cup of coffee."

"Help yourself. While you're at it, think about having a pair of seats not far from the fifty yard line. Eh?"

Smith had to pay his fine before springing for extravagances. Any extra cash he had would go to gas vouchers, if he could find them. "Can I talk to you for a minute?" he asked Ralph with a nod toward the stairs.

"What's up?" Ralph asked when they were out of earshot. "You want to score those tickets without the guys knowing?"

"Do you have any gas vouchers?"

"Sorry, nothing in that department. In fact, I'm looking for some myself. My lady wants to get back to the shore for another one of our romantic interludes. She'd be willing to juggle a schedule or two at the HAO of your choice for twenty gallons worth of paper."

Given that he was thirty gallons in the red, Smith had nothing to offer, not that he would have made the exchange in the first place. He learned his lesson with regard to breaking the rules of the Universal Coverage System.

"Timmy's fine," he said. "I'm just running short of gas myself."

"That's a shame," Ralph replied. "I mean about the gas, not Timmy. I hear your boy has an awesome swing."

"After some batting practice, he'll be one hundred percent," Smith finished.

Settling at his desk, Smith had every reason to expect that he would be reinstalled as team leader. His 1412 violations had been settled without adversely affecting Wexler Associates. Only the paperwork needed to catch up, which couldn't take longer than another day or two.

It wasn't to be. The week droned on with Smith doing nothing more important than shuffling through old train station plans in the company archives. He nagged Henny Geerman until she shot him a terse email about spending too much time in the human resources lobby. He dared to reply that there was no reason for him to attend Friday's wellness meeting. Henny's reply read like a regimental order.

"You will continue to attend all mandated treatment sessions until further notice. Unapproved absences are subject to a Section 1412 hearing."

The trouble with emails, Smith thought, was you couldn't crumple them up like old-fashioned memos and have the satisfaction of throwing them in the trash, which is exactly what he wanted to do with Geerman's reply. The delete button did not have the same stress-relieving impact, and Dr. Solorzano's sessions did nothing but aggravate him for the waste of time that they were.

Nonetheless, he showed up Friday night as scheduled. There was a guest speaker, an undertaker, who pitched the group on natural burial for themselves and their loved ones. At the end of his spiel, Solorzano had everyone form a circle for the final chant of the evening.

"Let me return to mother earth," he extolled.

"Let me return to mother earth," Smith repeated with the other attendees. He found it easier to join the asinine chorus than to remain quiet at the risk of being singled out for Solorzano's personal ministrations. However, he was unwilling to stand there with his eyes closed as everyone else did.

"Let me be free from the grief of earthly mortality."

"Let me be free from the grief of earthly mortality."

"Death is not a loss," Solorzano said.

This was not a new phrase, but for some reason Smith couldn't say it. He heard voices around him say the words, mimicking Dr. Solorzano's emphasis on "not."

"I embrace death's release," came next.

Infuriated by the meeting's absurdity, Smith felt the urge to punch the man next to him for squeezing his hand to the beat of the chant. Was the guy a moron? Death may or may not be a release of some sort, Smith thought, but it was very much a loss. Any claim otherwise was an inherent contradiction, like saying an empty bucket was full.

On the other side of the circle Smith noticed a man looking directly at him. He wore the fierce expression of someone in no mood for Dr. Solorzano's rapturous paradoxes. Smith offered a nod of recognition and received one in return. Glancing at the faces around him, he saw that they stood alone among the believers. Fortunately for the two of them, the meeting came to a close with the final refrain.

"By accepting death, I am free."

Smith broke loose from the grip of his fellow attendees and turned for the door like a kid on his way to recess. His escape was cut short by a command from Dr. Solorzano.

"Bob! Hold on a second."

His desire to ignore the request was overcome by his fear of having to answer for it in Henny Geerman's office. He turned back, hoping the train would be late the way it had been the week before.

"There is someone who wants to speak to you," Solorzano said.

Smith's immediate thought was to the guy who looked as unhappy as he felt about the meetings, but Solorzano ushered him into a side room where a cheerful young man noisily chewed gum as he tapped out a jazz beat with an E-tablet stylus.

"Hi," he said cheerfully after finishing his imaginary song. "I'm Gary Bell."

At this point, Dr. Solorzano excused himself, shutting the door on the way out.

"What can I do for you?" Smith asked.

"Just a couple questions," answered Bell, smacking out a few beats before continuing. "I work for the Medical Service Bureau. We're a sort of blanket agency. We fill in the gaps where regular law enforcement doesn't have traditional authority."

Harkening back to his 1412 hearing, Smith said, "I've heard that."

"Mostly I investigate situations and make a report to the enforcement division, which makes a decision to take action or not."

Feeling his time slipping away, Smith said, "If this is about my 1412 hearing, I've already sent a check for the fine."

"No. That's all wrapped up."

"I wish it was," Smith countered. "I shouldn't be here, and I should have my regular job back. Do you know when that paperwork is going to catch up or the computers are going to connect?"

"I don't know anything about those particulars, just that your 1412 file is satisfied. I'm here about something else."

"Which is?"

Now Bell took out a digital tablet and read from the screen. "During a recent meeting here you spoke with a woman named Leslie Clacher."

Instantly, Smith recalled Phil's admonition that he say nothing about the *Salvare*. He remembered thinking the man was paranoid, that no one would care where he went to get his chemotherapy. Even if they did, they wouldn't waste time tracking him down to make a federal case of it. What difference did it make if he paid for treatment outside the system? In a way it was better in that it made room for someone else.

Yet, here he was being questioned by a guy too young to be an experienced detective but with all the authority to act as one. Bell's cheerful manner did nothing to put Smith at ease. He guarded his answers not to protect Phil but to save himself from another fine or garnishing of his fuel ration.

"She introduced herself as Leslie," he said. "She never used her last name."

"You spoke to her and then outside you talked with an older male, her husband, Phillip Clacher."

There must be cameras on the side of the building, Smith thought. Or maybe Solorzano had people in the group keeping an eye on the others. Or worst of all, Phil and Leslie might be bait in a trap to catch people going to the *Salvare*.

"Phil seemed like a nice guy," Smith said.

"I never met him. Did Mr. Clacher discuss his health condition with you?"

"I'm not a doctor. Why would he discuss a health condition with me?" Smith returned to avoid answering the question directly.

Bell started tapping his stylus, a tic that betrayed his nervousness. Despite his obvious agitation, he stayed on point. "Did he discuss his health condition with you?"

Realizing how quickly the subject of Bell's inquiry could change from Phil to himself, Smith confidently feigned ignorance by using the truth. He said, "I don't know anything about his health."

"You did talk to him," Bell pushed.

"I talked to him and Leslie."

More tapping preceded a new angle on the original question. "Did Clacher mention anything about his recovery?"

"Recovery from what?"

The tapping stopped, and Bell swallowed his gum like a frog gulping a fly. "I ask the questions. You answer them." This statement should have come from the bad cop in the good cop bad cop scenario, but Bell was alone. He had to play both sides, except that his bad cop wasn't so bad despite lowering his voice an octave.

"I understand," Smith said, detesting the haughtiness of this punk. He had the urge to ask for identification, but before he had the chance, Bell got back on track.

"What did you talk about?"

Again, Smith employed the truth. "We talked about our wellness meetings."

"What about them?"

"How we couldn't wait for them to be over."

"Why can't you wait for them to be over?"

"Because they're a complete waste of my time."

"Is that what Clacher said?"

"That's what I said," Smith replied, boldly looking at his watch to see if he might make the train.

"Have somewhere to be?" Bell wanted to know again slipping into bad cop mode.

"Yes. I have a wife and son at home. I'd like to be on the 9 PM train if it's all the same to you."

"We'll see," Bell told him. "You talked about the wellness meetings. What else?"

"That's about it."

"How long did your conversation last?"

"Not long."

"Not long enough to remember a single other thing you talked about?"

"I was in a hurry to make the train that night, too."

"You sound like a busy man. Do you have any idea why Leslie did not attend the meeting tonight?"

"I can't imagine why she wasn't here," Smith answered. He couldn't imagine because he didn't have to. He knew why she wasn't holding hands and chanting like a numbskull, or listening to an undertaker hawk the latest fashion in human burial. Nonetheless, he had no inclination to share this information with Bell.

"Leslie Clacher was not here because there have been a

number of spontaneous recoveries recently," Bell explained. "Her husband is one of them."

"Good for him."

"Maybe it wasn't spontaneous. Maybe he received treatment outside the Universal Coverage System."

"What if he did?" Smith asked, breaking the rule about who asked the questions.

"That depends," Bell replied. "Let's say he received treatment at an unlicensed facility."

"There aren't any," Smith interjected.

"You haven't seen the ads for the *Salvare*?"

"I've seen them."

"Then you are aware of an unlicensed facility," Bell said, pleased at catching Smith. "Assume Mr. Clacher was treated aboard the *Salvare*. If he got approval, there's no problem."

"What if he didn't get approval?"

"A client can't have it both ways. Either they receive all services and treatment in the system or none. The Healthcare Administration Authority grants permission to go outside the system. Anyone can apply. By doing so, they stay within the bounds of the law."

"Why would anyone do that when they'll lose all future benefits?"

"That's the point. We can't have people playing both sides off the middle, cherry picking what they want when it's convenient."

"Maybe they're just trying to get help," Smith said.

"Think about it this way," Bell prodded. "It's like the President's slogan: ONE FOR ALL. If everyone went outside the system, there wouldn't be one system for all, would there?"

Smith left that question in the air between them.

"We're not out to make anyone into a criminal," Bell said, changing to an affable good cop. "This is a civil matter. It's their responsibility to do the right thing and support the system, which provides so much to so many. You don't want to go back to the bad old days when the insurance companies ruled your life do you?"

Again Smith remained silent.

"Good. We understand each other."

"Just so I know, what happens to someone who gets treatment outside the system without approval?"

"You've been through a 1412 hearing. Do I have to go over that with you?"

Smith shook his head.

"Check Section 2018 of the UCM for the rest of the details," Bell clarified. "Until then, let me inform you that withholding information from a federal official with regard to fraud committed against the Universal Coverage System is a crime."

With his goofy manner and stilted phraseology, Bell reminded Smith of the cop at the fuel depot. Sure, he possessed the authority of a federal agent and a badge to prove it. He might even carry a gun to match his cute electronic accessory. He was still too young, too smug, and too smart by half to do the job of a serious detective. If he wanted to do it well, Smith thought, he should study Detective Elroy's methods in a few episodes of *On The Prowl*. Now there was a guy who knew how to ask the questions.

In that frame of mind, Smith said, "I'm going to go home and review the Universal Coverage Manual tonight, Mr. Bell. You see, my son needs some follow up care, and I'm going to make sure he gets it so that I don't have to waste another minute here talking about death."

Having swallowed his gum and failed to intimidate his suspect, Bell put away his digital tablet and tucked his stylus behind his ear.

"No need to be grumpy. I have a job to do, questions to ask, reports to file. You're on my list, and now I can check you off it."

"Yeah," Smith said, "and one last question. Are there any licensed facilities outside of Universal Coverage?"

"None."

CHAPTER
SEVENTEEN

OF THE CURRENT THINGS THAT AGGRAVATED HIM MOST, Smith's encounter with Gary Bell topped the list. That the government employed such investigators to compile reports on people like Phil Clacher was a waste of time and tax money. Wouldn't it be better to hire a few more doctors and nurses? He appreciated the need to enforce the rules, but if a guy wanted to take his chances at an unlicensed facility, that was his problem.

Or was it?

If the doctors there botched a procedure, or gave the wrong medication, or committed some other act of malpractice, and Phil returned to his regular health district, his self-created disaster would be everyone's burden to bear. It would be that much more expensive, having been made worse by the likes of some unaccredited bunch of freelancers.

Then again, he and Hannah hadn't supported a program that would send the gendarmes in pursuit of medical scofflaws. The goal was that everyone had coverage, that they could get treatment regardless of their income or status, that they wouldn't be left at the door while someone with cash in hand stepped over them. Sure, there was a need to prevent abuse, but why wasn't anyone looking into Rieser and Plant? That was a direct assault on the public and at the hands of government employees no less. It didn't take Detective Elroy to figure it out either. Anyone with his eyes open could catch those two red-handed.

Smith might have dwelled on the issue more, or been chafed by the delay in getting his job back, or irritated by having to ride the FART for a month straight. But all these things fell into perspective, becoming lost among the little things of life where they belonged. This happened because he had every reason to forget about the whole affair. Henny Geerman informed him he was foundation team leader again. The computers were finally in synch according to the company's human resources director. The foundation team celebrated with a lunchtime feast that was sure to put everyone on the wrong side of the scale come the next quarterly health review.

While gratified to have his job back, Smith was delighted to skip the Friday evening wellness meetings. No more holding hands or chanting or sitting on the floor. Rather, he was where he belonged, watching the Media Moguls win three out of every four games they played, thanks to their star player who had a GP appointment scheduled for three months hence.

At the end of August, Mark Wexler called another company-wide meeting to announce that Central West was back on track, the entire project passed its audit with flying colors, and the infrastructure teams had better get busy with their intercity rail designs.

"This President means business," Wexler said. "He wants train stations that makes the ones in Europe look like outhouses."

The room issued a round of supporting applause.

"We're going to schedule a first shovel ceremony soon," Wexler was saying. "Afterward, I want to show the President a range of station designs not only for Philadelphia, but other major cities. We can't think of ourselves as a local firm anymore. We're going to reach out to the entire country and mop up as much stimulus money as we can."

The normally reserved engineers, designers, and estimators burst into football stadium cheers. Smith himself surrendered to the moment, shouting the way he did at Timmy's games. And why not? He paid his 1412 fine, had a ten-gallon gas voucher in his pocket, and was making plans to move into Philadelphia as soon as possible so the vouchers would become irrelevant.

Neither Smith nor Hannah discussed the possibility of leaving the suburbs with their son. Timmy was attached to his teammates and Coach Dolante, relationships his parents did not want to disrupt, especially in the middle of a winning season. However, between the two of them, they acknowledged that it was best for all of them to head for the city. When the time was right, Smith would break the news that Timmy could look forward to playing in a new stadium.

While Smith cheered with his colleagues, he saved some of his excitement for Timmy's game tonight. The Moguls faced the West Chester Cougars at 7 PM. The Southeast Pennsylvania Energy Management Board granted a special variance to turn on the lights, which was bound to give the game a big league feel.

Loyal fan that he was, Smith bolted from work at the end of the day. He coasted into Delaware County Fuel Depot Number 3 to purchase his first gasoline in over a month. Thanks to his frugal use of the vehicle he had an eighth of a tank remaining or about three gallons. Clutching his voucher, he remembered that he promised Timmy a trip to the Valley Fair Ice Cream Shop, win or lose, after the game.

Halfway across the parking lot, he met four grumbling customers retreating to their cars. A guy wearing painter's pants stopped short and spoke with Smith.

"Can you give me a ride to Ridley Park?" he asked.

"I guess," Smith replied. "Did your car break down?"

"Yeah, it's a fuel problem," the painter said. "As in there is none."

"You ran out?"

"No, the depot ran out."

"There's no gas here?" Smith blurted.

"That's why I'm looking for a ride."

"But I have a voucher."

The guy pulled one out of his pocket, stretched it between his two hands, and said, "So do I. You know what you can wipe with it, don't you?"

"There has to be gas," Smith shot back. "The system issues vouchers when ..."

"Forget it," the painter moaned. "Let's get out of here."

They turned around and headed toward Smith's pickup.

"I can't believe this," the painter complained as he pulled his door closed. "Didn't they up our allotments this month?"

Smith remembered the President himself making the announcement on television.

"I mean, how can they issue vouchers if they don't have gas?"

"Must be a supply chain error," Smith offered, using the same words he'd used when speaking to Mr. Fetterman about his medication.

"Yeah, right," mocked the painter. "You know what I think? I think those guys working the depot skim a few gallons off the top every day."

"That's not fair," Smith put in. "You don't know they're thieves."

"Come on. Think about it."

Smith actually took a few seconds to ponder the possibility then said, "I don't think they could get away with it. Every gallon is tracked from the time it arrives until the time it is pumped into your car. They'd come up short if they were stealing."

"And what happened today?" asked the painter.

"You don't know that they ran out because someone was stealing. A delivery truck might have broken down."

"Here's how they get away with it. They rig the pump so instead of getting ten gallons, you get nine and a half. I was thinking my car's mileage was off, but now I've changed my mind."

"The county weights and measures department certifies the pumps every year," Smith told him. A man used to arrive at his dad's gas station with a special measuring bottle for this exact purpose.

"They used to," the painter corrected him. "Fueling depots are federal facilities now with their own inspectors. All it would take is a few bucks in his pocket to look the other way. They might even reset the pump before he showed up."

"It's possible," Smith admitted, "but unlikely."

"Either way, we have no gas and that's a big problem. How am I going to get to the job tomorrow?"

"You can't take the bus?"

"How many five gallon pails of ceiling white can you carry onto a bus?"

One more reason to move into the city, Smith thought, knowing it was the best way to avoid the painter's dilemma.

"Thanks for the ride," the painter said when Smith stopped at his corner. "I'd be happy to discount any painting work you need done."

"I'll keep that in mind," Smith replied, but he had no plans to touch up his house in Cliffwood. He intended to sell it as is, where is, if he could find a buyer. This problem was minor compared to telling Timmy that they wouldn't be headed for ice cream with the other kids.

For his part, Timmy gobbled his supper wearing his uniform and stepped onto the front lawn for some batting practice. Not having a pitcher, he imagined the ball coming in, swung the bat, and darted for first base, which was just past the mailbox. Arriving ahead of the phantom outfielder's throw, he stared down the block, wondering how Joey Anzalone was doing on his team. Coach Dolante hadn't said anything about the "city teams" as the Philadelphia groups were known. It didn't matter. Whoever pitched for Joey's team would be gaping at the sky when Timmy hit the ball over his head, past Joey's outstretched glove, and over the wall.

He ran across the street, to the opposite corner where he figured second base should be, and kept going to the corner of the driveway for third, then back to the lawn for home plate.

Reaching for his bat, he felt that flutter again, the one that had vexed him during his game against the Titans. He leaned on the bat for a few seconds to catch his breath. Feeling better, he swung a few more times, ran the bases, and then headed inside to get his dad. He was ready to play the game.

They arrived at the field in plenty of time. Timmy hopped out of the truck leaving Smith to park it alone. Hannah went on an apartment-hunting mission bearing several private listings she'd found on the Internet. Smith would have liked to sit with her at the game but knew it was best if she winnowed down the real estate list on her own. He trusted her to find a good value in a decent neighborhood. Under cover of visiting her friends, Timmy was none the wiser.

As he approached the stands, Smith searched for Mr. Fetterman. No one stood at the right field wall — his usual viewing spot. Smith staked out the area, greeting other regular fans as they made their way to the bleachers. By the time the teams took to the field, Mr. Fetterman still hadn't appeared, which concerned him because he hadn't seen the old guy in more than a month. Smith decided to remain where he was in case Mr. Fetterman appeared.

"Play ball!" shouted the umpire.

The pitcher for the Cougars had a devastating curve ball. The Moguls suffered through the first four innings with too many strikeouts and a few mistakes in the outfield, allowing the Cougars a two-nothing lead. Timmy managed to hit a single, but the same pitcher who faked out his fellow batters, managed to keep him pinned to the base. The kid seemed to have eyes in the back of his head because every time Timmy stretched his lead, he hurled the ball to the first baseman. Several times, Timmy had to dive under the throw or be hit by it.

In the top of the fifth, the Moguls rallied. Timmy caught a line drive, immediately launched the ball to the second baseman, who caught a Cougar runner in a pickle with the help of the first baseman. The Cougar's next batter struck out, giving the Moguls an opportunity to step up to the plate with confidence.

This they did. The first batter read the pitcher's intentions correctly and landed a double. The next kid struck out but not without a good fight. Then came another single. It was Timmy's turn, and the crowd stamped their feet for him. They wanted a home run, and their energy flowed into Timmy's shoulders as he loosened up before taking his stance. It was time to teach this pitcher a lesson, to show him that it took more than a few fancy throws to retire a champion. He stared straight into the other kid's eyes, watched him wind up, and instinctively shifted his weight to put some power behind the bat.

The crowd jumped to their feet only to release a collective groan as the umpire shouted, "Foul!"

A foul is a strike by another name, Coach Dolante always said. Timmy used those words to channel more determination. Looking for Mr. Fetterman, he spotted his dad by the wall. He risked a smile as he thought it would be quite a feat to hit a fly right out there to where his dad was standing. Wouldn't that be something? They'd probably put the picture on the Internet. DAD CATCHES SON'S HOME RUN, would be the headline. How many kids could say they did that? None that Timmy knew. He could be the first and the definition of a champion was the guy who finished first.

Flexing his knees, he expected to feel the flutter again, but it didn't come. In fact, he felt as solid as a telephone pole, ready to drive that ball into oblivion. The pitcher tossed the ball to his second baseman a few times, an obvious ploy to unsettle the batter he faced. The opposite occurred as Timmy focused more intently.

As confident as Timmy was, Smith experienced a level of anxiety he hadn't felt since he first asked Hannah out. He wanted his son to hit that homer. At the same time, he worried that the boy might strike out. It wasn't the end of the world; there were still several innings to go, but with two men on base, now was the perfect time to take the lead.

Smith saw the ball fly from the pitcher's hand. It seemed that Timmy simultaneously swung the bat. There had been a brief instant between the two events, and during that split second, the ambulance departed the field for another game on the other side of town. When he spoke with the ambulance crew a few weeks ago about their early departures, Smith learned that there was a shortage of emergency medical technicians. Therefore, they had to split their time among the various sporting events on any particular night.

The driver tapped his siren the way he always did when he steered out of the parking lot. The sound distracted no one because the whack of solid hickory connecting with a three-inch sphere of leather-covered yarn had everyone's attention.

Timmy's aim was a little to the left, which sent the ball on a trajectory more toward center field than over his father's head. He dropped the bat on his way to first, aware that Coach Dolante hollered for him to run faster. There was no need to hurry. The crowd's whooping told him the ball was gone. He jogged around first, kept his head down past second and third, but couldn't resist a glance toward his dad on his way to home plate.

Smith saluted Timmy with both arms in the air. His boy had done it, put the team ahead, and did so on the second pitch. Modest champion that he was, Timmy responded with a gentle thumbs-up as he placed his foot on the plate.

"That a boy, Timmy!" Coach Dolante called.

Timmy turned back toward the stands. He absorbed their adulation, which made his chest feel full, like an inflating balloon. It was a strange feeling, one that left him light-headed but happy and content. He practiced the way his coach taught him to. He watched the pros and studied every move they made. The payoff: he was on his way to being one of them.

Suddenly, someone started taking photos of him. They were close, too, because the flash nearly blinded him. Wanting to look his best, he smiled. More flashes followed, smaller ones. He held up his hand for them to stop.

All at once he couldn't remember where he was going. His arms turned incredibly heavy and he lost track of where his feet were. He stumbled, tilted forward, and dropped onto the grass near the on deck circle.

CHAPTER
EIGHTEEN

THE PEOPLE AROUND SMITH PUT UP THEIR HANDS for high-fives and congratulated him on his son's achievement. He blushed with pride, responding that the game wasn't over yet.

"Oh, yeah, it is," someone replied. "The Moguls are going to run all over them."

"You got it!" another fan agreed. "We're gonna see your boy playing for the Phillies one day."

"I'll bet college scouts have their eyes on him already."

The crowd settled down in anticipation of the next play, but the batter stood off to the side with his teammates. The visiting team gathered into a knot with their coach.

"Let's go Moguls!" a guy near Smith shouted.

Instead of standing behind the catcher, the umpire kneeled beside Coach Dolante. Both of them leaned over Timmy who lay on his back. Two of the bigger kids moved closer only to be waved away by Dolante.

"That's your boy, isn't it?" the guy next to Smith asked, pointing.

Without pausing to answer, Smith sprinted as if trying to outrun a line drive. He slid to a stop, nearly colliding with the umpire who at that moment was standing up.

"Get the ambulance!" yelled Dolante.

"Is he breathing?" Smith asked.

"Barely," Dolante replied then turned his head toward the umpire and added, "The ambulance, Marty!"

"It left already."

"Damn. Call 911."

"I'll get my pickup," Smith said and bolted toward the parking lot.

Fans for both teams sat muttering about the poor kid laid out down there. They'd heard about Timmy's previous collapse, but chalked it up to growing pains or the pressure of being a star player. After some weeks off, he was back on the field, hitting better than ever, stealing bases at whim, and leading his team toward a championship. Now it looked like he was down for the count, something they prayed would never happen to their own children.

Dolante draped Timmy over his shoulder in a fireman's carry and hustled off the field, led by several Moguls who cleared the way. He saw kids knocked out cold by line drives, break their legs while sliding into home plate, and a broken jaw thanks to a carelessly tossed bat. As shocking as those injuries were, they were to be expected in the course of a game. Timmy, on the other hand, seemed perfectly fine, which made his sudden collapse all the more unnerving. It was like walking through a minefield; you just never knew when it was going to happen.

Smith bounced over the curb, bringing his pickup to a halt as close to the field as he could. Someone yanked open the passenger door and Dolante eased Timmy onto the seat.

"Go!" Dolante urged even though his own door was not quite closed. It slammed hard at his side, the panel bruising his arm in the process.

A few years ago, Media General replaced several smaller hospitals in the area. A massive complex, it towered over the west side of town, at least six stories taller than the next largest building. It was only a short drive from the Moguls' field at normal speeds. Smith covered the distance in record time by running every stop sign and traffic light.

The Emergency Entrance fronted Baltimore Pike, fed by a sweeping drive wide enough to accommodate a tractor-trailer. Smith used every inch as the pickup slewed sideways, stopping with a bump against the curb. He looked down at his son who was unconscious and the color of old paste.

"Lead the way," Dolante said. "I'll bring Timmy."

Just inside the entrance door Smith found a uniformed guard. "I need help!" he blurted. "My son's ..."

"Chester General or Springfield Memorial," the guard said. He held out a sheet of paper that Smith reflexively accepted.

"This is an emergency. My son has a heart problem. He's collapsed."

"Follow the instructions I gave you," the guard said.

"Where are the doctors? The nurses? I need someone right now!"

"There's no one here."

"What are you talking about?"

"There's a temporary service suspension. It's supposed to end in three hours."

Smith glanced about the space and saw that no one else was there. For a second he thought he'd somehow come to the wrong place, that in his panic he'd stopped at a shuttered grocery store or something, but there were signs on the wall, one in four languages, pointing to various medical departments.

Just then, Dolante passed through the automatic doors carrying Timmy in his arms. "He's coming around," he said. "Where should I put him?"

"Take him to Chester General or Springfield Memorial," the guard said loud enough to be heard outside.

"I want a doctor right now!" Smith yelled. "Go get someone!"

"Only essential staff are here, and they're all busy upstairs," the guard responded flatly.

"Is he kidding?" Dolante wanted to know.

Smith advanced on the guard. He was going to find a doctor if it meant kicking down every door in the building.

"Stop!" the guard commanded. "I'm ordering you out of here."

Smith darted around his adversary, plunged through a pair of swinging doors, and put on speed. The clatter of the guard's utility belt spurred him on. Turning the first corner, he slipped on the floor, banged off the wall, and kept going. The hallway doubled back, leading past a row of examination rooms and administrative desks, none of which contained a single human being. There was a fish tank positioned high on a counter. The angelfish inside stared sideways through the glass. A second later, the guard was upon him.

"There's no one here," Smith said, gulping air.

"That's what I told you."

Smith bolted again. This time, the guard let him go.

"He's breathing better," Dolante said as Smith returned to his side.

"We have to get out of here."

"I don't think he's out of the woods, Bob."

"Give him to me," Smith said, slipping his arms under Timmy's body. He'd never felt someone as cold as his son was at that moment. Lifting him was like picking up a sack of chilled twigs. Timmy let out a groan, which provided a welcome sign that he hadn't expired.

"Do you know where Chester General is?" Smith asked.

"Sure," Dolante responded.

"Good. You drive."

Just outside the Emergency Room doors, Timmy moaned again, convulsed, and spewed a stream of vomit.

"Careful he doesn't choke," warned Dolante.

Smith squatted down, tilting Timmy's head to the side to make sure he could breathe. Worried that he wouldn't get to Chester General in time, Smith rose and headed for the pickup.

"Who's gonna clean up this puke?" the guard called after them.

"We'll get there," Dolante said taking the wheel.

"Don't kill us on the way," Smith advised.

"Hang on to your boy. He's my best player."

Smith noticed the low fuel light flashing before Dolante, who was too busy looking out for other traffic. He thought back to earlier that afternoon, when he'd given the painter a ride. What if he'd wasted the gas he needed to get to the hospital on a simple act of generosity?

Dolante spotted the low fuel light. "Damn!"

"The fuel depot ran out today," Smith told him. The depot guard's voice flashed through his mind. Never before had he paid attention to how many security personnel seemed to be about. They wore different uniforms and answered to various agencies. Nonetheless, they stood by at fuel depots, train stations, health administration offices, and hospitals. His father never had anyone looking over his place. Nor had there been anyone more menacing than a semi-retired school teacher who tended the reception desk when Timmy was born at Riddle Memorial Hospital.

Looking down, Smith saw that Timmy's eyes were open.

"Something stinks," he said.

Smith couldn't hold back a smile. "We're on our way to the hospital."

"What smells?"

"You threw up, champ," Dolante said.

Timmy insisted on entering Chester General on his own two feet, but after only a few steps, he pitched over just as he did at the game. Smith caught him in time, wrenching his own back in the process. Dolante took the boy's feet and helped lug him into the building.

A triage nurse named Bonnie met them.

"He's got a heart problem," Smith said.

"At his age?" Bonnie queried.

Having gotten his thoughts together on the drive there, Smith explained, "The cardiologist who reviewed his case thought it might be arrhythmia."

"Put him down here," she said with a wave to an empty gurney. She put her stethoscope to Timmy's chest, closing her eyes as she listened.

Only then did Smith notice the goings on around him. On a row of plastic chairs against the wall sat a dozen or more people with various wounds. Blood leaked through bandages, eyes swelled shut behind bruises and icepacks, broken limbs hung from slings and temporary splints. Feeling as if he stepped into a military field hospital, Smith glanced at his own son, who showed nothing worse than grass stains on his uniform, yet desperately needed help like everyone else.

"He barely has a pulse. I'm taking him in," nurse Bonnie said. She took out her digital tablet. "Give me both your names."

Snapping out of a daze, Smith asked, "Is he okay?"

"I'll let you know. What's his name?"

"Timmy. Timothy Smith. I'm his father, Robert."

"Step back Mr. Smith." With that, she released the gurney's brakes and shoved it forward. Before passing out of sight, she reminded Smith to check in with reception.

"Wait a second," he called.

Only the creaking doors replied to his plea.

"He's in good hands now," Dolante said, pulling his champ's dad back a few yards. "I'm just glad we didn't run out of gas."

Of all the things he was supposed to be doing, Smith called Hannah first. The line rang eight times before switching to her voicemail. He closed his phone, paced back and forth across the hallway a few times, and tried again. The second bounce to her voicemail was not a surprise. He gave up and headed toward the reception desk.

A beefy guy who held one bloody hand in another stepped in front of him. "What makes you so special?"

"Excuse me?" Smith asked.

"You rush in here and get treated like a king while the rest of us have to hang out like we're waiting for the paint to dry. You pay that nurse off or what?"

"My son has a heart problem," Smith explained. "He needs immediate treatment."

"Yeah, we all heard you. Like if I don't get these fingers sewn back on I might as well throw them in the trash. Just tell me how much you paid so I can keep all my pieces."

"I don't know what you're talking about," Smith said and moved around the guy.

"Why didn't you fly him out to that ship? You know, the floating hospital that advertises on TV. Don't they do heart jobs?"

Ignoring the comment, Smith stepped up to the receptionist and reached for his Universal Coverage Card. It was his new card that he handed to the woman on the other side of the counter. "Universal Coverage: The best care possible," it read across the top.

"Is there something you can do for that guy with the bleeding hand?" Smith said.

The receptionist accepted his card and replied, "With Media General closed, we're doing all we can to keep up."

"Why are they closed?"

The receptionist ignored his question. The printer beside her desk gave birth to another file that would soon join its two dozen siblings on her desk.

"How can an emergency room be closed?" Smith wondered aloud.

He spent the better part of an hour filling in blanks on forms he'd seen before. This annoyed him because in the HAO, not to mention Henny Geerman's office, the computers seemed to be able to talk to one another very efficiently. At least the monotony relieved him of greater worries, but only for a while. Twice he approached the receptionist for an update on Timmy. Both times, other patients or relatives beat him to the window. He stood by resignedly, reminded by Coach Dolante that no news was good news. If the worst had occurred, someone would have told him. He retreated to the far end of the waiting room, where he propped himself against the wall for lack of an available seat.

During the hour he waited, Smith learned the names of the Care Delivery Specialists who repeatedly entered the room to collect people like him. Each of them inspired a moment's hope in the eyes of those waiting. The one who ultimately came for him was Joan Foster. She wore the white coat of a doctor that flowed behind her like a cape as they wound their way to the elevator.

"It's probably faster if we take the stairs," she said offhandedly after pushing the call button.

Used to climbing the ten floors at the Wexler building, Smith replied, "Let's go. I want to see my son."

"Relax, Mr. Smith," Foster said. "Your son is resting quietly. You'll be seeing him in a few minutes."

Those few minutes of agony evaporated when Smith arrived at Timmy's side. He felt an uncontrollable urge to laugh, as if the past several months had been an extended prank. Smith alone smiled at that moment. He gazed down at his son, not sure what to do.

Timmy blinked lethargically and forced a swallow. He almost confessed that he'd not felt well on many occasions leading up to this one. How much would this episode cost his dad? Would it be another trip to that ugly building where a smartalec fined him more money than it cost to buy every starting player a new glove? Would it be less gas? Would his dad have to be away every Friday night at some meeting he complained about to mom? The weight of this guilt hurt more than the ache in his chest, which felt ten times worse than when Brett Long plowed into him on his way to third that time.

Either way, Timmy knew something was wrong. Whatever it was, more than the baseball season was in trouble. He alternately felt as if he might black out or throw up. That these feelings came and went without warning terrified him. He was used to being strong, to charging at first base like an angry bull. Presently, he could hardly feel his feet. How could he be a champion without two good feet? He almost apologized to his dad for going down in the middle of the game, but his dad was already talking to someone.

Smith realized that his son lay on a gurney near the end of a hallway instead of in a room. He faced Foster and replied, "What's my son doing in the hall?"

"Non-critical patients are held in common areas until a space becomes available in a bay suite." For her upbeat tone, she might have been hosting a tea party.

"I want to speak with his doctor."

"Dr. Cooke is on the way," Foster responded. She looked past Smith and added, "Okay, that space is available."

Turning to the left, Smith saw an orderly struggling to wheel a bed through the last door in the corridor. After four tries and much banging against the doorframe, he finally exited and proceeded past Smith, Foster, and Timmy. A white sheet covered all but one hand of the person on the bed.

Timmy remembered an episode of *On The Prowl* in which a body lay on the ground just like the one that passed him now. If the sheet covered their face, it meant they were dead, and Timmy had no doubt that whomever it was going by, they were headed for the morgue. That's where Detective Elroy went to check the bodies for clues.

Smith saw Timmy pressing his eyes closed to stave off the tears. The giddy relief that he'd felt earlier was replaced with a building rage that left him squeezing the stainless steel rail flanking Timmy's bed. Still, he didn't want to further upset his son.

"Your homer put the Moguls in the lead," he said.

Timmy's eyes snapped open. "Did we win?"

"I'm sure of it," Smith answered.

"Here we go," Foster interjected.

The orderly who passed them parked his previous charge not ten feet down the hall. He strolled up to Timmy's bed, stomped the brake loose, and heaved it toward that last door on the left. Thanks to Smith's assistance Timmy entered the suite easier than the previous resident departed.

Inside there was only one place for the bed to go: immediately to the right, just past a lavatory from which came the sound of trickling water. Seven other beds filled the room along with several empty chairs and one occupied by a tiny, wrinkled woman.

"You have to leave," the orderly told her unceremoniously.

The woman sobbed, but didn't move.

"Can you tell her?" the orderly asked Foster.

"I'm a Care Delivery Specialist," Foster replied. "Call Loss Coping. Grieving relatives are their job."

"They don't answer," remarked the orderly.

"Try again."

Just then Dr. Cooke entered the room. In an instant he surveyed the scene and moved to the woman's side. "I'm sorry, Mrs. Weller," he said.

"He's with the angels now," she wheezed.

"He is," Cooke soothed her. "Do you need a ride home?"

Weller coughed. "That damn bus got me here. I suppose it will get me home."

"It's getting late," Cooke reminded her.

"Dr. Cooke," Foster put in. "We have another case waiting."

Glaring at Foster, the doctor said, "I'm not blind, Ms. Foster." He then helped Mrs. Weller to her feet, ushered her to the door, and released her to find the bus after she insisted that no more aid was necessary.

"I was born before everyone had a car so it's nothing strange to do without one now," were Mrs. Weller's last words on the subject.

Cooke greeted Smith with a handshake and then focused his attention on Timmy. "By the looks of your uniform, you play hard," he said.

Timmy managed half a grin. "Not today," he replied.

"Let's see what we can do to get you back in the game. Okay?"

"Okay."

Smith, Dr. Cooke, and CDS Foster stepped into the hallway for a conference. Cooke wasted no time getting to the point.

"Your son has cardiac arrhythmia, Mr. Smith. The signals that control the muscles of his heart get out of synch, and then his heart doesn't work properly. The lack of blood flow causes Timmy to pass out. I won't sugarcoat it. This is a very serious condition. If not addressed, it can be fatal."

"As young as he is?" Smith protested weakly.

"When I first started practicing medicine there was a famous basketball player who died on the court. This isn't a question of age or conditioning. The problem is the electrical system."

"You said it can be addressed."

"My recommendation is that Timmy receive a pacemaker."

"A pacemaker?" Smith repeated. The last time he heard this

term was when Mr. Porter, the owner of a '92 Chevy Caprice, pulled into his father's station, opened his shirt, and showed him the surgery scar on his chest.

"The pacemaker senses when the heart's rhythm is out of synch. It sends a signal to the muscles, which gets them working properly again."

"I knew a man with one a long time ago."

"The good news is that a pacemaker does the job in nearly every case. Once in a while you change the battery, and you're good to go."

"Great," Smith said, relieved to hear there was a reliable solution to his son's problem.

"Timmy is going to stay with us for a few days to monitor his condition. When I spoke with him earlier he said he wasn't experiencing any other symptoms, but I suspect that this has been getting worse."

Foster said, "Patient statements are to be taken at face value."

"Excuse me, Ms. Foster. I have a couple of sons myself. They would never admit to something that kept them out of a championship season."

"The data suggests ..."

Cooke cut her off. "When was the last time you saw a pro athlete cry on TV?"

Smith broke the tension by saying, "If a pacemaker is what Timmy needs, let's get it done."

"Your son's name will be in the pool for this procedure," Foster informed him.

"The pool?"

"The pool is the list of patients waiting for a category of procedures, in this case, cardiac surgery ..." Cooke began to explain.

"You are the doctor," Foster steamed. "I'm the Care Delivery Specialist. I would appreciate it if you would allow me to clarify any of the patient's questions regarding the sequence of treatment."

"By all means," Cooke said with a wave of his hand.

"As Dr. Cooke mentioned," Foster went on, "a request for Cardiac Care Level 3 will be entered into the system. Depending upon current demands, his treatment will be scheduled."

"Current demands?" questioned Smith. "How does that work?"

"It's a lottery," Cooke said.

"Dr. Cooke!" fumed Foster. "The selection system generates an unbiased order for the sequencing of treatment. Many factors determine the order."

His education included numerous courses in advanced mathematics, a few of which taught Smith that an unbiased order of sequencing meant the same thing as a lottery. "Are you telling me you hold a random drawing to pick who's next in the operating room?" he asked.

"No, Mr. Smith. You misunderstood me," Foster said, "Your son's …"

"That's exactly what she's saying," Dr. Cooke cut in.

"Doctor, you are very close to an official censure," Foster said, then added to Smith, "It's not a lottery. It's the only fair way to ensure equal care for all clients."

"Hold on," Smith said. "Dr. Cooke, tell me the truth, how is my son doing?"

Cooke folded his arms. "Your son's heart has suffered some minor damage from today's attack. He's a strong kid, no doubt about it, but an acute episode of severe arrhythmia could result in the worst."

"In other words he needs this pacemaker right away," Smith translated.

"That's my professional opinion."

"Now, Ms. Foster, by whatever means you work these things out, how long until a spot opens up for Timmy?"

"There's no way for me to answer that question," Foster replied.

"Look," the doctor said to Smith, "There are eight hundred thirty-four people in the pool right now for Cardiac Care Level 3. I happen to be one of four doctors who treat the patients in this pool. Some procedures take longer than others, which means on average we take care of twelve patients every day. Do the math and you'll have your answer."

Smith did the math. "Timmy may have to wait two and a half months," he concluded.

"That's if we work every day, Mr. Smith. Even doctors need a day off once in a while. It could be four to five months."

"Dr. Cooke has failed to mention that your son may be treated as early as next week," Foster said. "The system automatically reprioritizes in the case of emergencies and for various other reasons."

His first thought was to his reinstated status on a CGP and how it might help Timmy's chances.

"That's right," Dr. Cooke was saying, "Mrs. Weller's husband was waiting for a reprioritization but his emergency came first."

"You were warned, Cooke. I'm writing you up," Foster declared.

"Use this," the doctor replied and handed her his pen.

CHAPTER NINETEEN

"CAN'T I GO HOME, DAD?"

"Dr. Cooke wants to keep an eye on you."

A technician entered the room, attached sensors to Timmy's chest, and plugged the wires into an electrocardiograph. "All set," she said cheerfully when the display came to life. Each beat of Timmy's heart scrolled across the screen.

When the technician left, Timmy pointed at the monitor, saying, "See that, I'm better again, dad. I'll be good for a couple of months."

Knowing this was not the case, Smith replied, "It's getting late. Go to sleep, and I'll be back in the morning."

Timmy had outgrown the bogeyman, but his father understood the boy's fear of remaining in a darkened room with people who might have escaped Doctor Frankenstein's laboratory. Sight of Mr. Weller's dead hand peeking out from under the sheet stuck in his mind, as he guessed it did Timmy's. Couldn't the orderly have been a bit more careful?

As difficult as it was to leave his son, the steady pulse on the heart monitor reassured Smith that for the time being his boy was doing well. No doubt the monitor had an alarm that would alert the nurses if something went wrong.

On the way home, Smith didn't pass a single moving vehicle, though he was too distracted to notice. Knowing the pickup was dangerously low on fuel, Coach Dolante asked to be let off on Baltimore Pike. "I'll walk the rest of the way home," he said.

"You sure?" Smith asked.

"Keep going before you run out," Dolante said as he closed the door. "Let me know how Timmy makes out."

"I'll do that," Smith finished and released the brake.

The pickup didn't let him down. He drove all the way to Cliffwood's gate before the engine stuttered twice and died. Coasting another hundred yards, Smith stopped three driveways short of his own, where Hannah's SUV sat at an odd angel.

Why hadn't she answered her phone? Smith wondered as he entered the house.

The clock on the microwave displayed eight minutes after eleven. Smith passed through the living room, expecting to find Hannah seated at the edge of the couch watching the news the way she did every night. No one was there.

"Hannah!" he called.

Getting no reply, he headed for the bedroom, where he

found her sprawled on the bed and most of her clothes in a pile on the floor.

"Wake up, honey," Smith said, shaking her shoulder.

With a groan and a weak slap, Hannah rolled over.

Smith needed no more evidence than her condition to know she'd been drinking with her girlfriends, probably too much to have driven home.

"Alright. Alright!" she protested.

Hannah made her way to the bathroom, explaining that she found a great apartment, a brand new two-bedroom, freshly re-habbed, only two blocks from the subway. It was important that they move fast before someone else leased it.

"I celebrated with Claudia," she said returning to the bed-room with a glass of water and her eyes barely open.

This news Smith accepted with a snort. His pickup was out of gas, Timmy needed a pacemaker, and Hannah celebrated find-ing an apartment they could not afford. Again, Smith felt that uncontrollable urge to laugh.

Hannah must have sensed it, or maybe he had a goofy look on his face. Either way, she asked, "What's so funny?"

"Nothing's funny," Smith answered. "Timmy collapsed on the field tonight. He's in Chester General."

"Why didn't you call me?"

"I did."

"Oh my god," Hannah sighed. She fumbled through her clothes to the purse at the bottom of the pile and pulled out her cell. "I turned my phone off when I went in the restaurant with Claudia and forgot to turn it back on."

Seeing his wife rushing to get dressed, Smith said, "Take your time, visiting hours are over."

Hannah sat down next to Smith. "Did you say Chester?"

"The Media emergency room was closed," Smith answered.

"Closed? Emergency rooms don't close."

"Apparently they do."

"What did the doctor say?" Hannah asked, the full weight of the predicament shrinking her beside Smith.

"He's in the pool for a pacemaker."

"In the pool for a pacemaker," Hannah repeated. "Who said that?"

"The care delivery specialist," Smith told his wife.

"We have to get him to a cardiologist right away."

Her sense of urgency impressed Smith in an odd way. She was the one who accused him of overreacting, of not trusting the doctor who initially examined Timmy, and now she was ready to pull out all the stops, which as he knew better than her, was a complete waste of time. The people at the Health Administration District Office were not the kind of genies who granted wishes. They entered data and regurgitated the computer's results. What had Care Administration Specialist Ledsoe said, something about the demands of the system at the time? Dr. Cooke explained that demand in plain language: 834 patients needed care akin to what Timmy required. If things went according to the numbers, the Media Moguls' best batter would get his pacemaker sometime in the next five months.

Then Smith considered there was another set of numbers at work. He calculated the odds that Timmy would have another attack before the pacemaker. The result frightened him. What were the chances that Timmy would bounce back the way he had in the past? That equation he couldn't solve. How much more damage could his heart sustain? He couldn't figure that one either.

There was one person Smith knew who might be able to

answer those questions. He went to the kitchen and dialed the number.

"I'd rather not ride with him," Hannah announced from the kitchen table.

It was the next morning and Smith had just unplugged his cell phone from the charger. He said to his wife, "Doctor Ben knows the cardiologist who saw Timmy last night."

"Why didn't you tell him we'd meet him there?"

"My truck is out of gas. Your SUV has barely enough to get you to the fuel depot and that assumes they have any fuel to sell."

"You told him that?"

Hannah's vanity seemed cute when they dated. Despite her claims to the contrary, appearances mattered and vulnerability was something never to be admitted. She was chic in her intentionally distressed clothing worn in college. As their careers provided more wealth, she slowly morphed into an understated fashion queen who always seemed to have the right outfit for every occasion along with all the appropriate accessories. Nowhere was this more obvious than at the Little League games she attended. Nonchalant glances of other men fell upon her as much as toward the sound of the bat, attention she coyly denied while simultaneously acknowledging it with a faint smile. She flirted with Josh, too, on those mornings when he arrived early for their commute. Strangely, Smith had taken pride in having Hannah as his own. He saw her not so much as a trophy but as a secret treasure. Though at this moment, he understood the burden of her façade.

And he was in no mood to carry it.

"You can take the bus if you want to, but Doctor Ben is on

his way, and I'm going with him."

"I can't wait until we live in the city," Hannah moaned, "and don't have to catch a ride with farmers."

Upon arrival at Chester General, a uniformed security guard greeted them from the visitor reception desk. He accepted Smith's Universal Coverage Card and driver's license along with the same two forms of identification from Hannah. Doctor Ben offered his visiting physician certificate.

"Wait a minute," the guard said after logging everyone's name into the computer. "You two are fine, but he's from 128. You got a waiver to work here, Doc?"

"I'm providing special consultation on this case," Doctor Ben said. "Check under Section 578 of the UC Code. Visiting physicians are permitted to attend to those cases which may provide additional educational opportunities to other medical personnel."

"Oh, sorry," the guard said. "Just doing my job."

"Of course you are," Ben said.

Supplied with visitor badges the three of them took the stairs to the eighth floor and Timmy's room. On the way up, Smith asked about Section 578, as he didn't remember what it said.

"I don't give a damn what Section 578 says," Doctor Ben told him. "These fools just need an answer to their stupid questions. They don't know the difference between the right ones and the wrong ones so long as you give them any one."

"Great," Hannah whispered to herself. "Just great."

Neither Smith nor Doctor Ben paid her any mind.

"Dad!" Timmy called when his parents entered. His heart monitor soared to one hundred fourteen.

"Settle down," Smith said.

"How are you doing?" Hannah cooed as she circled to the other side of the bed.

"Ready to go home," Timmy told his mother. A night's rest had done him immeasurable good. Gone was the weary heaviness of his limbs and with it the nausea. It took him several hours to get to sleep, what with the other people in the room wheezing, sputtering, and even farting. He told himself he'd been captured by an evil villain who locked him deep in the bowels of an old factory. His own team was going to break him out soon enough. All he had to do was rest up for the fight that would inevitably come when they arrived. Here they were: his mom, his dad, and Doctor Ben, too.

He sensed his mom's nervousness, which at first struck him as unfounded. He was strong again, willing to race anyone down the stairs. His dad looked worried, too. Maybe they came to tell him something bad about his heart. As for Doctor Ben's presence, he didn't know quite what to make of that. He'd only met the man once before but had liked him immediately. He gave off an air of confident authority, which Timmy admired the way he did the pros who stepped to the plate, took a few practice swings, and then hit one out of the park.

Thus, with three people staring at him and seven others lying in semi-consciousness, Timmy began to feel insecure. Was he going to end up like his roommates? I'm too young for that, he told himself.

Then Dr. Cooke entered the room. "Good to see you, Ben," he said, extending his hand. "How's life on the farm?"

"Got the mill running," Ben replied.

"Headed back in time are you?"

"Not without a fight."

To Timmy, Dr. Cooke then said, "You look like you're ready

to play in the World Series."

"My coach thinks so," Timmy replied.

"I'm going to talk to your parents for a few minutes. Then we'll be back in to work out how to get you on the starting roster."

Timmy liked the sound of that. He gave his mom a stage wink the way any self-respecting action hero would right before he escaped the clutches of his enemy.

In the hall, Dr. Cooke checked his watch and scanned the area. He wasn't part of Timmy's imaginary plot; he had genuine cause for concern. "Foster will be here in a few minutes," he said.

"She's the CDS?" Doctor Ben asked.

"Yes, and a very enthusiastic one," Cooke noted. "She's already set Timmy's care plan in stone."

"What does that mean?" Smith queried.

"Your son is going home," Cooke answered.

"Today?"

"Monday, middle of the morning."

"That soon?" Hannah queried.

"Let me explain," Cooke said evenly. "I tried to keep him here, but Foster checked your Citizen Health Profile and discovered that you're from District 117. She has to get Timmy out of here before Rule 72 kicks in."

"Rule 72 is slang," Doctor Ben interjected, "for the period after which a patient, sorry, a 'client' as we're supposed to call them, becomes a cost to the district where they are hospitalized."

"What difference does it make?" Smith wanted to know.

"Each district only has so many resources: doctors, nurses, operating rooms, drugs. If someone from one district is treated in another it takes away from that district's ability to serve their own people," Cooke said.

"More importantly," Doctor Ben added, "their costs go up while their theoretical population remains the same. This is a no-no in the zero-sum realm of Universal Coverage. Budgets are meant to be enforced. Each CDS gets a rating based upon how they manage their designated resources."

"That's idiotic," Smith huffed.

"Unfortunately, that's the way it is," Cooke observed. "Foster's arranged for Timmy to be discharged to your care until his surgery can be scheduled in your district."

"What if he has another attack?" Hannah inquired.

"Rush him to the emergency room," Cooke advised.

What if it's closed? Smith wanted to ask, but Doctor Ben was already speaking.

"Joel, what's your take on Timmy?"

"He needs the pacemaker, Ben. He seems to be stable at present, but his heart rhythm fluctuates enough that he's at risk for more than a fainting spell."

No urge to laugh came over Smith this time. Rather, he felt compelled to beg Dr. Cooke to do whatever it took to get Timmy that pacemaker as soon as possible. At the same time, he knew this was futile. It wasn't up to the doctor; Timmy's course was to be determined by the demands of the system, which would be interpreted by someone like Care Administration Specialist Ledsoe in consultation with the Care Delivery Specialist at Media General or whatever facility the system remanded him to. All the while, Timmy's heart ticked away the minutes that may be either the beginning of the rest of his life or the end to what his life had been.

"You with us?" Doctor Ben asked Smith.

Smith forced a nod; Hannah blinked.

"There is an alternative," Cooke said. "Two of my classmates from med-school work at another facility. I would trust these guys with my own kid."

"I'd be grateful for the referral," Smith said.

"If you want to do it the right way," continued Cooke, "you'll have to apply ..."

"Why waste the time?" Ben cut in.

Shaking his head, Cooke replied, "He has to know what he's getting into."

"Where do I find your friends?" asked Smith.

Ben answered, "Aboard a ship."

"*Salvare?*"

"Without approval you face fines in the thousands of dollars," continued Dr. Cooke. "With approval you'll be cut off from Universal Coverage."

"I've been told as much," Smith said.

The sound of CDS Foster's heels coming down the hallway prevented any further discussion.

"Mr. Smith!" she called. "I have good news for you."

"Finally," Hannah muttered, "someone with a real solution has arrived."

"YOU'RE AN ENGINEER. YOU CAN HANDLE IT."

CHAPTER TWENTY

IT WAS ONLY AFTER CDS FOSTER HAD BEEN SPEAKING with him for ten minutes that Smith realized how wonderful his life had been. No crisis interrupted the steady attainment of his desires. He grew up in pleasant circumstances with only the usual discipline of a serious father, and that training enabled him to apply himself in college as well as at work. The smooth ascent of his career satisfied his material wants and sustained his standard of living even in the face of the country's economic disaster. He recognized the challenge, adapted accordingly, and overcame minor inconveniences like riding the FART or waiting for an Energy Conservation Event to end. Along the way, he obtained enough wisdom to know that everything was cyclical. He positioned himself to ride the wave up or pause for another one to come in. Only the ignorant slid backward.

However, CDS Foster was explaining, in an entirely too cheerful manner, how much better Timmy would do at home. She was the game show host sidekick touting the benefits of his prize package: Timmy would be in familiar surroundings, among people he knew, and able to watch whatever he wanted on television. While this was true, it did nothing to solve his problem. That she refused to address the real issue is what triggered Smith's self-evaluation. Aside of his parents' deaths, which were both normal and expected, he'd never faced a problem he couldn't work out with a bit of study or a few more dollars. In rare cases, he called a specific expert for help. And he got it.

CDS Foster, unlike his colleagues, wasn't offering much. She did have an automatic external defibrillator, which he was to take with him. "You have to give it back," she said, "after you're re-established in your home district. They'll give you another one, and then you can return this unit to us here. Be sure they log it in the system and give you a receipt."

He nodded to the cadence of her words like some dolt at a rock concert. Simultaneously, he considered that he knew nothing about using such a piece of medical equipment. He noticed Hannah staring at the bright yellow box with the red stripes on the side. He wondered if she would be able to use it, or if she would panic and freeze.

"The AED instructions are inside the case," CDS Foster said with a wave. "You just pop it open, follow the steps one by one, and you're back in synch like the Rockettes on stage at Radio City Music Hall."

What a relief! Smith thought. I'll just hook my boy up to the shock box for a quick jolt and he'll be back in the game. Couldn't he at least be provided with some training the way he'd been given for CPR as a Boy Scout? According to Foster, there was no need.

"Besides," she said with a flicker of her pen atop a carbonless form, "I'm overtime on this case so as it is. Your District 117 CDS can help you out if you really feel it's necessary."

Overtime? Just how long was each case to take? And who figured that out? Was it a good idea for amateurs to be sending umpteen thousand volts to a child's heart?

These questions tormented Smith, a punishment that seemed appropriate for a guy who skated through so many years with nothing more painful than a stubbed toe.

"You're an engineer," Hannah was saying. "You can handle it."

"Don't forget to be here at least half an hour before discharge time on Monday," Foster reminded them.

At last he found his voice and said, "I'd like to transfer him directly to another hospital."

"I've checked the CER on this. Timmy will be fine at home until his Cardiac Level 3 Care Plan can be implemented."

"What's CER?"

"Comparative Effectiveness Research," Foster explained. "One of the benefits of the Universal Coverage System is the amount of data it collects. We correlate each case with its treatment and results. That way we can more efficiently allocate system resources for the best outcome."

Again, Smith's knowledge of mathematics kicked in. He considered that two data points, a 1 and a 10 for example, could be averaged to five. However, there was no five in the set. Was this how Universal Coverage worked? Was it set up to handle the 5's with no consideration for the 1's and the 10's?

"Care doesn't end in the hospital," Foster was saying. "If you'll sign here that you have been thoroughly and properly briefed, I can be on my way."

"How do I go about getting Timmy a new CDS and getting him into a group for the pacemaker?"

"A quick stop at your District Admin Office. Give them all the paperwork you have and they'll take care of the rest. It's that easy."

Hardly, he wanted to tell her.

"Sorry to rush you, Mr. Smith, but I need you to sign this form. I have other clients waiting. We're completely swamped."

"Thank you so much for all your help," Hannah said.

"No problem," Foster returned. "Just doing my job."

Smith scribbled on the form because he knew Foster had a rote answer for every one of his questions.

"Bye, Timmy," Foster said with the kind of smile the Penner sisters used to give Smith from the wheel of their matching Camaros after they filled their tanks at his father's station. Foster left the room without so much as a second look at Doctor Ben who had been going from bed to bed, speaking with each of the other patients.

Luckily for Hannah, Doctor Ben's pickup was the crew cab variety. She sat in the back, on the passenger side, pressing herself against the door to be as far away from the driver's position as possible. Smith rode in the forward seat without ceremony or an explanation for Hannah's petty behavior, which he was sure Doctor Ben had detected.

Before they left Timmy's room, Doctor Ben took a minute to listen to his heart. Hannah stood by looking as if she swallowed a rotten pickle.

"You'll be out of here on Monday," Doctor Ben said to

Timmy, "if not sooner."

"Yeah. I'll be ready for Friday's game," Timmy told him. "Are you gonna watch us play?"

"That sounds like fun."

"We'll all be there," Hannah chimed in.

"You, too, mom?" Timmy asked hopefully.

Suddenly Hannah lost her voice. She opened her mouth to speak then closed it into a flat smile.

Coming to the rescue, Smith said, "See you tomorrow, champ."

Doctor Ben had barely stopped in front of the house before Hannah hopped out. She rushed to the door, rummaged through her purse, and finally found her keys. Without waiting for her husband, she burst in, slamming the door behind her.

"Thanks for everything," Smith said to Doctor Ben. "I apologize for Hannah. She's ..."

"Forget it," Ben cut in. "Let's go for a ride." He didn't wait for Smith to agree. He simply turned around in the middle of the empty street.

Half an hour later they stared at the spinning wheel of Doctor Ben's mill. Gone were the broken timbers, scattered stones, and the Amish who presumably removed them. The building bore the fit and finish of a new structure. Every mortared joint was tight, every window clean. The recently graded road gave the impression that a farmer might arrive at any moment with a wagon full of corn ready for grinding. Incongruously, a single light bulb, encased in a protective fixture, hung over the doorway. It glowed a dim yellow, which Smith found odd given that it was the middle of the day and there were no wires leading to the building.

"Follow me," Doctor Ben said as he started for the door.

Inside, Smith discovered the source of the light bulb's electricity. A series of belts connected the waterwheel's main shaft to a small generator mounted in the center of the room where the grinding stones normally would have been. A distribution panel with meters showing the generator's output and voltage stood against the far wall.

"The Amish put this together for you?" Smith asked.

"Everything but the wires," Doctor Ben answered. "They're not much for electricity."

"I didn't think so," Smith reflected, moving closer to the system. "Nice and quiet."

"My Amish friends had no problem figuring out where to put the ball bearings," Ben said pointing toward the main shaft.

Indeed, the whole affair displayed the top-notch craftsmanship of a professional installation. Had he been on an inspection tour, Smith would have affixed his engineer's seal to the official certificate. The only thing missing was a government permit for the system. He knew better than to ask Ben if he had obtained one for it or for dredging the pond above.

Doctor Ben peeked over his glasses at the meters on the electrical panel. "Ahhh, perfect," he said then turned to Smith. "There's one more thing."

Marvin waited for them atop the step to the back door of thehouse. He darted inside, leading them into the kitchen where he went straight for his water bowl.

"Fancy cat, he doesn't like to lap from the stream," Doctor Ben commented. "Would you like a drink yourself?"

Smith shook his head.

"Apple?"

"Thanks," Smith said and helped himself to one on the table.

The fruit was crisp and delicious.

"Amazing how long these will keep in a cool cellar," Ben said, taking one into his hand. "I think I'll do an experiment to see just how many months they'll last."

"I should be getting home," Smith said. "Hannah's not dealing well with Timmy's problem."

"This way."

Instead of exiting the house, Doctor Ben led Smith down a short hallway to the front room, which had been arranged as a library.

"Mr. Fetterman!" Smith exclaimed.

"What's left of him," Fetterman replied groggily. He put aside a book that straddled his lap and struggled to get up.

"We missed you at the games," Smith said, chagrined that he hadn't taken the time to look up the man over the past month.

Fetterman's eyes gleamed with his usual pluck, but the rest of his body was a wreck. By the color and drawn texture of his skin, not to mention the foul odor, Smith knew that Timmy's most loyal fan suffered from a disease not likely to have a positive outcome.

"How's your boy? Ben tells me he's back on the disabled list," Fetterman said, standing atop shaky legs.

"He'll be fine. What about you?"

"My liver's about finished, but I'm as good as can be expected for a guy who got I double-E'd."

"What does that mean?"

"Tell him, Ben."

"Remember when Foster mentioned Comparative Effectiveness Research?"

Smith nodded.

"The CER data creates a ratio: the cost of more treatment

divided by the number of extra years a patient might live if he receives that care. If the ratio is too high, you get an I double-E rating. It stands for Imminent Expiration Event. After that you get pain management only."

"Which doesn't always work," Fetterman groaned.

Horrified, Smith countered, "It can't be that simple."

"You're looking at it," Fetterman said. "Ben keeps me comfortable with hard cider and whatever extra pills he filches. It doesn't look like I'll make another one of Timmy's games. I wish they were on the radio. I remember listening to baseball several nights a week. I'd be in my shop, cutting a suit or sewing up a cuff. The game would be on. One time I wasted three yards of the best worsted wool over a bases loaded strikeout. What was the name of that guy?"

None of Dr. Solorzano's chanting had prepared Smith for the idea of Mr. Fetterman not standing at the outfield wall. Nor had it convinced him to accept the freedom of death, whether it be a man as old as Mr. Fetterman or a boy as young as Timmy. In the presence of someone obviously close to passing on, Smith felt helpless and frustrated that more couldn't be done. At the same time, he realized that this was the way he should feel. He shouldn't be chanting mindlessly about death's release or shouting for joy that he was free. It was natural to despair, to mourn.

Then there was the issue of the I double-E.

"Let me talk to those people at the Health Administration Office," Smith offered.

"No point," Fetterman told him. "You get one appeal. I had mine the last time I saw you and Timmy there. They ruled against me."

"One appeal? Even convicted murders get more than that."

"They probably get better doctors, too. No offense, Ben."

No one laughed at the remark.

Mr. Fetterman straightened his shirt, looked to Smith, and said, "I'm an expert tailor and an authority on baseball. Your boy's going to make the World Series. I know it."

Smith certainly hoped this prediction would come true.

"Ben says he's building a little field out here in the lawn. Has that Amish gang coming back next week. Maybe Timmy and some of his pals could show up and play a few innings for their number one fan before he goes to the stadium in the sky."

"You can count on it," Smith said, though after a look from Doctor Ben, sensed that Fetterman was not going to live to see it.

Doctor Ben drove smoothly. The roads leading from the Thorpe Estate rambled across handsome scenery. Smith recalled that his father taught him to drive on these country lanes. His first time at the wheel had been early one Sunday morning when few other cars were about. It was the same now, only not because people were sleeping in or getting ready for church.

They rounded a bend, coming upon the same Rural Beautification Crew Smith had passed earlier in the summer. One of the trucks was nearly full of utility poles. A crane was positioned to lower another one onto the truck. At the behest of the flagman, they stopped to stay clear of the action. Looking forward, Smith saw that no power lines stretched into the distance.

"I'm doing what I can to get to the future," Doctor Ben said.

Not taking his meaning and upset about Mr. Fetterman, Smith remained silent. He watched the crew clamber atop the truck in order to unhook the pole they had just set on the pile.

"They're taking down the power lines," Smith said, starting to make sense of it all.

"Rural beautification," Doctor Ben clarified.

"That's why you rebuilt the mill and put in a generator."

"One of the reasons."

"It's not easy to live in the country, is it?"

"No more difficult than the suburbs."

Smith thought about that until the flagman waved them through. "It's another I double-E," he muttered.

Doctor Ben eased his foot on the accelerator. Neither a smile nor a frown marked his face. He said nothing to his passenger for the remainder of the journey, not until they passed through the gate at Cliffwood and parked in front of his house.

At last, he said, "Find a ship."

Hannah didn't want to hear it. Her solution was to make a fuss at the HAO.

"I'll go there myself," she huffed, pointing a finger over her shoulder. "This is a boy's life not a case of the sniffles. As soon as that's clear, we'll see some action."

Amen! Smith almost shouted. Not being a religious man, he kept the sentiment to himself. After Hannah waited several hours for the opportunity to unleash her tirade, she would discover that no amount of browbeating was going to motivate the HAO people. Instead, she would find out whose birthday it was and who got the presents and who didn't. Eventually, an appointment would be made, but only when the computer spit it into someone's lap.

"Honey," Smith said, "I'm going to call Lynn and ask her how to get to the *Salvare*."

"That's crazy," Hannah shot back. "That place doesn't even have a license!"

"Dr. Cooke's friends from med-school work there. He highly recommended them. Doctor Ben feels the same way."

"What makes him an authority?" demanded Hannah.

Taking a breath first, Smith said, "Don't you remember how we found your obstetrician? The one who delivered Timmy?"

"My obstetrician? What does she have to do with this?"

"She was recommended by my mom's doctor who had retired."

Hannah didn't get the point. With a roll of her hands she urged her husband to get to it.

"Doctor Ben came to my father's gas station at least twice a week as did a bunch of his patients."

"Because he hung out with the grease monkeys he knows what's best for Timmy?"

"He didn't hang out," Smith explained. "He bought gas there. Everyone knew he was a doctor and asked him about whatever ailed them. He always had a kind word or the name of another doctor for them to call."

"Spreading around the fees to his golf buddies," Hannah scoffed.

"Helping people get to the right person," countered Smith.

She shook her head. "Is this some kind of loyalty thing, Bob? Do you think you owe this Doctor Ben character something because he bought gas from your dad?"

"That's ridiculous. Before we had computers collating Comparative Effectiveness Data, people were free to refer each other based on their own experience."

"Let's not ignore what else Dr. Cooke told us," Hannah said. "If you take Timmy to that ship, we'll be cut off from Universal Coverage. We'll be fined thousands of dollars. Is that what you want to happen?"

"No," admitted Smith.

"Then we have to follow the system."

"Hannah, you're in for a challenge at the HAO."

"I'm going to help you, Bob. We're going to work together to get Timmy whatever he needs. The best possible care, remember?"

"That's what we're getting," Smith said, "a defibrillator instead of a pacemaker."

"Which is a great start," Hannah finished.

Upon hearing this, Smith realized that more than Hannah's cooperation, he needed two things: transportation and money.

CHAPTER
TWENTY-ONE

ALONE IN HIS HOME OFFICE, Smith flipped through his address book, searching for Lynn's phone number. He came to Ralph's first. Staring at the entry, he took a moment to reconsider his plan, always a good policy in engineering and life. With nothing to lose, he decided it was worth a call.

"Boss!" Ralph answered. "Not like you to ring me on the weekend. Hope you're not looking for any gas vouchers."

"No, something else," Smith replied.

"Good, because I hear they're going to rework the system. The vouchers are going to be sent out every week instead of once a month. That's going to make it hard to trade them."

"I guess it will," Smith said. While he needed fuel for his

pickup, he thought maybe Ralph could arrange an appointment for Timmy. He asked, "How are things with your lady friend?"

"Awesome," Ralph replied. "We're catching a play tomorrow afternoon. It's not my kind of thing, but when she says jump, I say how high."

"Sounds like she has you in the harness."

"All the way to the barn," Ralph joked.

On the back of this positive news, Smith made his petition. "Do you think she could fix things for Timmy to get a pacemaker sometime soon?"

"Wow. A pacemaker? Kind of young for that, isn't he?"

"He's in Chester General now. They're sending him home on Monday. He was in the pool for a pacemaker, but now he has to start over in our district. It could be months."

"That's a shame," Ralph said. "Look, I know this is your boy, and we're friends and co-workers and all that, but she's going to need something for the effort."

Smith expected this, but what did he have to give? More important, what did she want?

Pre-empting the question, Ralph said, "She likes jewelry. Nothing too fancy. Stuff she can wear around without drawing attention."

Over the years, Smith purchased a few pieces of jewelry for Hannah. Naturally, it started with a diamond engagement ring. A gold necklace and matching bracelet marked their tenth anniversary. She rarely wore the set, preferring more stylish pieces she bought to accessorize her outfits. For a moment, Smith considered that giving up these extravagances was a small price to pay for Timmy to move up the list.

"You still there?" Ralph was asking.

"Yeah," Smith answered but let the phone slide a few inches

from his ear. On the wall beside him hung a framed stock certificate for 100 shares of Exxon-Mobil. It was the only one remaining from the pile his father bequeathed. How much was it
worth?

"You gotta give a little to get a little," Ralph said of the pro-
posed transaction.

Without another word, Smith calmly returned the handset
to its cradle. Give a little to get a little? Hocking his wife's jewelry! Trading away the last of his father's legacy! What the hell
was he thinking?

The President, when he had been a candidate, referred to
Universal Coverage as an investment. Smith remembered the
speech. "We have to invest today to provide coverage in the future. If we don't take these steps now, we are allowing disaster
to come our way." He hadn't said anything about giving a little
to get a little. It was all about investing, cost savings, efficiencies
and effectiveness. The word synergy came up plenty of times,
too, but nothing about giving a little to get a little.

Smith had followed the President's lead. Each week he made
his investment: twelve percent of his gross income. He didn't begrudge the deduction given its purpose. Or maybe he did. Previously Wexler Associates took only two hundred fifty dollars per
month, hardly twelve percent of his gross pay. There was also the
twenty dollar co-pay when he went to the doctor. Still, Smith
believed he was doing the right thing, contributing to a system
that took care of people less fortunate than he. In the event he
lost his job, he wouldn't lose his health insurance. It was provided by the government, so it followed him wherever he worked
or even if he didn't work at all.

As the President had said, "No one should be without the
best possible care."

Smith agreed. Hannah did, too. They rallied and campaigned and even protested when less ambitious politicians dragged their feet. This was done with the expectation that they would live in a better, less fretful future, one without the possibility of wiping out their savings, or taking away their home, or putting them in debt for the rest of their lives. They were upwardly mobile, and although they were healthy, knew how a devastating illness could wipe out everything they were about to earn. They were still living in the two-box apartment, but bigger things lie ahead. After all, they already had cell phones, cars, spring break excursions to the Caribbean, and recruiters from well-known corporations promising them salaries to pay for more. For what seemed like a small sacrifice, the President's proposal insulated them from the possibility of losing it all. Isn't that how insurance worked?

They tendered their votes and moved on, proud to have been a part of history.

More important, their dreams came true. Both Smith and Hannah enjoyed an ever-improving standard of living. Gone was the two-box apartment. Banished were the second-hand vehicles. In came the gadgets, appliances, and furniture that made life fun, easy, and glamorous. Out went the cheaper clothes, used books, and college dorm shenanigans. Friends accumulated and coalesced around a social schedule of dinner parties, nights on the town, and weekend mini vacations. Some debt entered the equation, but the payments were easily made. While they hadn't saved much, why worry? They were adults. Along came Timmy to prove it.

Now Smith sat in his handsome home office before a desk of polished cherry under a wrought iron lamp that once sprouted four sixty-watt bulbs. Presently, a single fluorescent element stuck out from one of the sockets like an ugly wart. Outside, not in his driveway, but a few blocks away, sat his pickup. It was old, dirty, and out of gas, a condition only slightly worse than Hannah's SUV, which was nearly so. His original friends in Cliffwood, including the sworn hold out Tony Anazalone, were gone. The last time he and Hannah held a dinner party, or attended one for that matter, had been two years ago. He might have to pawn some jewelry not for cash to bribe someone but to buy gas if it became available. Smith's social scene centered around Timmy's games, the way it should, but without those games he might have qualified for a monastery. Hannah continued to venture out with her girlfriends, and Smith didn't begrudge her the fun, but it had never been so expensive.

The phone rang. He stared past it at the framed stock certificate on the wall. Something happened between the time his father received his dividends and this day. Smith never envisioned he would face disaster without a penny saved or a dollar in reserve. Nor had he expected to lack the gasoline to go wherever he wanted. The idea that whatever he needed might not be at hand was an absolute impossibility.

This was not the future he'd anticipated nor the one he'd been promised. He wasn't supposed to be giving a little to get a little. He was supposed to have on demand care without ever seeing the bill. That's what Universal Coverage meant. That's what he voted for. That's what twelve percent of his pay bought.

Without a doubt, it paid for financial security. He wasn't flush with cash, but nor was he in danger of losing his house, his vehicles, or anything else. He hadn't so much as seen a bill for any of Timmy's checkups. But what it did not buy was the timely installation of his son's pacemaker, something he wanted more than anything else.

He picked up the phone. "Hello?"

"It's me, Ralph. My cell must have dropped our call. Did you come up with something good for my girl?"

"No," Smith answered.

"No? Oh, I get it. You need some time. No worries. I won't say anything to her now. I'll wait until I hear from you. That way I can sell it to her as a special surprise. How does that sound?"

It sounded pathetic to Smith, who conjured up a witty retort but let it fade inside his growing shame.

"Have a good weekend," he said, hanging up.

The only person who deserved the money was the doctor who implanted Timmy's pacemaker. Anyone else was nothing more than a parasite taking something for nothing. Smith was ready to part with any of his worldly possessions, and if he had to mortgage his soul to make Timmy well, he'd do that, too. Either way, he'd be damned if he peddled his wife's baubles for better odds against the sharks who ran the Universal Coverage pool. He would take his chances aboard the *Salvare*, where from what he heard, he would at least get his money's worth.

Cradling the phone again, he dialed Lynn's number.

According to Lynn, getting to the *Salvare* was easy.

"You meet the helicopter at the Cape May Airport. It leaves at ten o'clock. Let me give you the number to reserve a seat. I hope you can get one."

"There are that many people using the service?"

Lynn laughed and said, "I think they could fill a seven forty seven."

Smith heard the phone drop followed by Lynn's cursing.

"Sorry, the phone fell. You have a pencil ready?"

Smith jotted the number into his field notebook, the one he'd intended to use during site visits to Central West.

"When they ask you about the referral," she explained, "tell them Vonda Franzini gave it to you."

"She's a doctor?"

"She's my cousin's friend. The one I told you about."

Wasn't this exactly what he'd been telling Hannah, people referring each other to good doctors?

"I wish I had listened to you sooner," Smith said, ashamed at having previously chastised her on the same matter.

"And I wish I'd sent Rose there. She'd be with me today if I hadn't sat around waiting for approvals. By the way, I don't imagine you're going to apply for one from the Health Administration Authority."

Upon hearing this Smith recalled his interview with Investigator Bell and Dr. Cooke's warning. He considered the ramifications of utilizing *Salvare*'s services. Someone from the Medical Service Bureau, perhaps Gary Bell himself, might be asking questions at the Wexler Building or cornering Coach Dolante before a Moguls game. Fortunately, he'd told no one other than Hannah, and now Lynn, about his intentions.

"I don't think I have the time," he said.

"If the MSB comes calling, I'll tell them nothing," Lynn promised.

"I appreciate that," Smith told his co-worker. Given her years of sparring with Ralph, he had no fear that Lynn could outwit someone like Gary Bell. Nonetheless, he considered the MSB might be more proactive when it came to *Salvare*'s customers. He asked, "Does the MSB have someone at Cape May taking names?"

"The airport is private property now so the most they can do is hang around the gate. Too bad for them the government sold it off when general aviation collapsed. Otherwise they'd be on site taking your photo and writing fines. We'd be screwed then, wouldn't we?"

"Probably," Smith concurred.

"Drive carefully. I know Rose is looking out for you."

Again Smith felt the profound sorrow of loss that nearly overwhelmed him in the presence of Mr. Fetterman. The difference was that Lynn's sister had already died, while Mr. Fetterman lingered, and similarly, Timmy awaited life-saving treatment.

"I'm sorry, Lynn. It shouldn't be this way."

"Do what you have to do," she instructed. "Take care of your boy. Good luck."

Although the President said nothing about giving a little to get a little, Smith recalled that he often mentioned doing what had to be done. The President called upon the nation to break with the past, to give up outdated notions about how health-care was administrated, financed, and delivered. The country followed. It followed all the way to the point where Smith was doing what he had to do — circumventing the entire system by meeting a helicopter in the middle of the night to fly his son to a ship loitering outside the international boundary for a procedure that in his father's day was as routine as telling the man beside the pump to, "fill'er up."

Filling his tank was his next problem, but Smith would take them one at a time. First was the reservation on that helicopter. Carefully, he dialed the number.

The woman who answered might have been the receptionist at a first class hotel. Her polished tone and sincere disposition made it easy for Smith to convey his situation. She asked thoughtful questions, responded with genuine emotion when he told her Timmy was only eleven, and assured him that the cardiac department aboard *Salvare* was staffed with highly qualified doctors.

"There is only one problem, Mr. Smith," she said, "The flight on Monday night is fully booked."

"Tuesday?" Smith queried with his fingers crossed.

"That one, too. After that we're repositioning."

"Repositioning?"

"Moving the ship to avoid a hurricane that's brewing in the Caribbean. It's forecast to come our way. Our captain thinks it best to sail farther east until the storm passes."

Smith couldn't remember the last time he paid attention to the weather. Not since he had a project underway and then he tracked it by the hour in order to rework the schedule. Once Central West cranked up he would be paying closer attention.

"I do have an opening tomorrow, Sunday night. Would you like that one?"

"I'll take it," he said.

"About payment, Mr. Smith, we accept all major credit cards, and cash is always welcome."

Looking at the stock certificate on the wall, Smith told her, "I have it covered."

"THIS CONCLUDES THE BOARD'S RULING."

CHAPTER
TWENTY-TWO

WHILE HANNAH SLEPT SOUNDLY IN BED, Smith thumbed through his gas vouchers. The problem was he couldn't stuff the paper in the tank of his pickup. He needed the gasoline, and he needed it right away. His father's station was always open early on Sunday morning. Smith had frequently worked that shift because the sparse traffic gave him plenty of time to do his homework. Then, around noon, things picked up, when people were on their way to family lunches or a trip to the mall.

Unlike his father's station, Delaware County Fuel Depot Number 3 was closed on Sundays, as well as every federal and state holiday. The same schedule applied to all depots in the county. Therefore, his vouchers were useless, which is why Smith saw that it wore a collar. It looked healthy, too. Someone was feeding him. After a few sniffs, the dog allowed Smith to pat his head then rolled over for a belly rub.

"There you go," Smith whispered. "That feels good, doesn't it?"

"Snuggles!" someone shouted. "Snuggles!"

Smith flattened himself on the trail. Simultaneously, Snuggles poked his nose toward the call. In a flash of paws and tail, the dog bounded away, leaving Smith with his face atop a matt of damp leaves. He dragged himself behind a tree and peeked out for a look into the neighborhood. Snuggles' owner turned out to be Greg Elbert, who stood in his boxer shorts in the middle of the street.

Relieved, Smith decided to get the rest of his gas from his own area. The last thing he wanted was another barking dog to awaken some light sleeper. He settled for fifteen gallons, nearly three quarters of a tank in the pickup, and enough to get him to Cape May. He dared not start it. That he would do during daylight, when no one would suspect him of anything.

Before going to bed, he packed a satchel with some of Timmy's clothes and placed the defibrillator on top. This he took to the garage, where he hid it among his father's toolboxes.

"All set," he whispered.

Having exhausted himself stealing gas the night before, Smith slept in Sunday morning. Apparently, Hannah had been busy during those extra two hours.

"We're not going to visit Timmy today," she announced from behind the remains of her breakfast. "We have an appointment."

Only then did he notice the Universal Coverage Manual, or what was left of it, spread over the table the way his father used to read the newspaper. None of the pages were the ones he'd marked during his exploration of the volume. Like the good student she'd been at Penn, Hannah used different color highlighters to indicate important passages.

"We're leaving in half an hour," she said next. "Get cleaned up while I make you some toast."

"Tell me about this appointment," Smith insisted.

"We'll talk on the way to the train."

"The train? Where are we going?"

"To the city, where people take these things seriously," Hannah replied. "Go find some clothes."

Seated in the passenger seat of his wife's SUV, Smith received a terse lecture on Section 2622 of the UCM.

"Forget about Doctor Ben and the *Salvare*. There's no reason to screw up our lives when Universal Coverage has plenty to offer, including a method to deal with system errors."

"It was Dr. Cooke who said his colleagues could help Timmy," protested Smith.

"Yes, he did, and he also mentioned the fines if you get caught. Timmy is not going for treatment anywhere other than here where he belongs."

To think that I was out stealing gas for just that purpose, Smith thought.

"Are you listening?"

"I am."

"Good. Section 2622 explains the Directed Outcome Assessment and Review Board."

"Is that DOA for short?"

Hannah slammed the brakes and said, "If you're not going to take this seriously, I'll leave you here."

Deep down he wanted to walk back to Cliffwood, get his

pickup, and head to Chester General. With Timmy at his side, it would be a short hop over the Commodore Barry Bridge and a leisurely drive to Cape May. They might stop at a fruit stand or an ice cream shop the way he used to when his own father sought out the first picking of New Jersey sweet corn. If time allowed, they could have a look at the ocean. Finally, he would park the truck with the windows down in the salt breeze and watch for the lights of *Salvare's* helicopter.

"Section 2622," Hannah was saying, "explains your rights before the Board. It operates twenty-four hours a day, seven days a week, holidays included. I knew this system would take care of us."

"Are you sure about the hours?" Smith queried, thinking that like the fuel depots, Universal Coverage was a federal agency and subject to the same operating rules.

"Look, I'm telling you what the UCM says."

Yeah, he wanted to remind her, and our vouchers say that we're supposed to be able to get gas, too.

Hannah continued, "Each state has several boards. The nearest one for us is conveniently located in Philadelphia, where we're going to live as soon as this horror show is behind us. The purpose of the board is to provide additional direction to care providers in order to achieve the best outcome."

"I thought that's what the Care Delivery Specialists did," Smith commented.

"You're forgetting that this is a review board, Bob. They review the actions of the system and assess the current outcomes with the goal of achieving a better one, especially in certain cases."

"I didn't know," Smith said, pondering that maybe he'd stolen from his neighbors unnecessarily.

"After our appointment today, we're going to go back through the entire manual. I'll bet there's more good stuff in there."

"How did you get the appointment?"

"That's the best and easiest part. All I had to do was go to the Board's website where you enter the codes and the system assigns you a time and date."

"The codes?"

"Every sheet of paper from Timmy's admission to the Emergency Room the first time, to the second opinion, to his treatment by Dr. Cooke, has a series of codes along the bottom. The CDS puts them there based on their on-site interpretation. Anyway, that's what the Review Board's web page is looking for."

Smith wanted to ask why these codes had to be entered again if the CDS did so already. Why didn't the Universal Coverage System's computers automatically trigger a board review? His opportunity to inquire passed because a proud Hannah pulled into a parking space at the FART station and told him to gather all the paperwork off the back seat.

Hannah and Smith encountered neither the pandemonium of the emergency room, nor the stress of a wait at the HAO. Rather, they arrived at a modern building with a spacious lobby of polished marble and shiny stainless steel. The Great Seal of the United States of America hung on one wall. Another was emblazoned with, Universal Coverage, The Best Care Possible.

Once again, a series of checkpoints separated them from their final destination. There was the obligatory sign-in desk, then a pass through the metal detector, and another I.D. check before they got to the elevators. The guards operating these posts showed none of the contempt displayed by Rieser and Plant. These chaps were attentive, helpful, and personable. Smith wondered if there was something added to the water, which also reminded him that he'd eaten only two pieces of toast with a smudge of strawberry jam. His stomach protested but he wasn't about to ask where he might find some vending machine goodies, not with Hannah on the march.

He found her attitude inspirational. This was the woman he knew in college, the one who rose above the right crowd and the smart parties. She cared about important things and did more than sit around and complain about the status quo. She took action, bold steps, doing the kind of things that used to make headlines back when there were newspapers to print them.

Smith missed this side of his wife and wondered why she let it fade. He knew the answer. It was the same thing that drained his will to be more politically conscious. They were comfortable. They climbed far enough up the ladder to enjoy a well-deserved break. On that rung he remained because it was easy to justify. He couldn't miss work for a rally. He had a mortgage to pay. How could he attend organizational meetings when Timmy had games several evenings a week?

Plus, things were more automatic now thanks to America Serves America, the outings for which Timmy attended every month. What other cause was Smith to support? He'd done his part for college admission diversity, for immigrant rights, for bringing the troops home, for stopping the oil companies from polluting, for controlling executive pay, for making sure that everyone had healthcare.

On that final thought he paused.

He worked hard for Universal Coverage, literally rejoicing when it passed into law because he genuinely felt it would bring about the best outcome for the most people. It had pained him deeply to think of how many people suffered with substandard care simply because they didn't have the money to pay. As he sat outside Hearing Room 1520, in a row with two dozen other petitioners, he had to admit he was less than hopeful the system for which he had been an ardent supporter was going to deliver anything more than it already had for his son.

Both Smith and Hannah spun their heads as the door opened. A perky young woman, who could have been Hannah's twin in college, waved for them to enter.

"Here we go," Hannah said.

Inside they were treated to all the trappings of a fully furnished courtroom. Nine tall leather chairs stood behind a high bench complete with nine gavels should any of the board members wish to bring the attendees to order. Before this sat a narrow table for the stenographer's computer. A few paces away were two larger tables, like the kind normally used by the defense and the prosecution. Finally, a velvet rope separated several rows of visitor seats.

There was but a single thing amiss: no one was there. That is no one but the young lady who now ushered them to that narrow table with the computer on it.

"Take a seat," she said. "I'm Katie Stuart, your Assessment and Review Specialist for today."

Smith figured Stuart to be twenty-three at most. How could she have enough experience to be a specialist? Come to think of it, every person he'd met in the Universal Coverage System called themselves a specialist of one form or another. Everyone but the doctors. They seemed content with a one-word title.

"Let me have your D.O.A.R. authorization so we can get started."

From her chair Hannah stared out at the empty seats.

"You have an authorization, don't you?" Stuart prodded.

Hannah snapped out of her trance and asked, "Are we early?"

"No," Stuart replied with a smile. "You're right on time the way you're supposed to be. Thank goodness you are. We AR Specialists are only permitted to hold the proceedings for 11 minutes. If we don't log into the computer by then, you have to reapply."

"What about the board?"

"The clock is ticking, Mrs. Smith. Let's get logged in, then I'll explain how things work."

Hannah produced her Assessment and Review Board Authorization.

Stuart used a hand held scanner wired to her computer to read the barcode at the top of the page. After a few strokes on the keyboard, she said, "Look at that, it worked. Let's see what we have."

Bewildered by the process, Hannah glanced about the room. Smith sensed her unease and gave her forearm a reassuring squeeze. He was used to the unexpected when it came to the system.

Putting her hands together between her thighs, Stuart spun her chair to face the Smiths. "Timothy Smith," she began, "whom I assume is your dependent."

"He's my son," Hannah said.

"It's so great to see a boy embraced by a traditional family setting. It's not everyday I get those. Anyway, just to review, your son was seen by an emergency room physician who issued a diagnosis that was confirmed by a second opinion then contradicted at a cardiac review. Subsequently, Timothy went to a different emergency room." Stuart paused, screwed up her face, and muttered, "I wonder why that was?"

"The emergency room at Media General was closed," Smith put in.

"Oh, way out there in District 117. I remember it well. Wow, did we have a flood of complaints! My boss told me it was a resource realignment that left staff levels below the guidelines. There was nothing they could do but issue a temporary service suspension, which was better than providing substandard care at an understaffed facility."

"My son might have died," Smith reflected quietly.

This didn't register with Stuart. She proceeded with her review, saying, "CDS Foster has issued a release date of Monday for Timothy Smith. He is to be seen by a visiting physician to monitor the case until the CAS in District 117 schedules a Cardiac Care Level 3 slot for him. Do I have it right so far?"

Chronologically speaking, she did, and both Hannah and Smith nodded affirmatively.

"Great. Now that I know all the information given to the board is accurate, we're on to the next step, which is ... early this morning, Hannah Smith requested a D.O.A.R. Board hearing. Mrs. Smith believes care directives for her son may have adversely affected, or will in the future adversely affect the outcome of the case. The basis for this is the failure of CDS Foster to immediately transfer Timothy Smith to District 117, where his case originated and is expected to proceed, along with the temporary inconvenience of Media General's service suspension."

"That's correct," Hannah affirmed. "She should have immediately sent Timmy to District 117, where my husband tried to take him to Media General, which, because it was closed, created this problem in the first place."

"Okay. Let's see what the board has to say."

Upon hearing this, the Smiths assumed there would be a

slight delay while the board was seated in order for the actual hearing to begin. They sat back in their chairs, exchanged a look and a sigh, and waited.

Katie Stuart wasted no time. She typed a few lines into her computer, stabbed the return key twice, and held her hand out for the pages coming from the printer. She handed one each to Smith and Hannah, keeping the final copy for herself.

She cleared her throat gently and read, "It is the opinion of the Southeastern Pennsylvania Directed Outcome Assessment and Review Board that ..."

"Hold on," Hannah interjected. "Where is the board?"

"The board, Mrs. Smith? What do you mean?"

"The people who sit in those chairs up there."

"They only meet once a month or as requested by the Universal Coverage Director."

"Then how can you be reading their opinion?" Hannah asked, not hiding her contempt.

"Because the computer gave it to me," Stuart replied.

"The computer gave it to you?"

Bristling at Hannah's tone, Stuart said, "Yes, Mrs. Smith, the computer. This morning you entered the data into the Board's system on your own computer, which fed it to the board's computer via the Internet. Remember?"

"I remember that very clearly, Miss Stuart, and I also remember printing out an authorization for a hearing, not for a computer to crunch some numbers and spit out a canned response to be read to me by you."

Smith knew it would be only a moment before Hannah was on her feet. He pushed his chair back a few inches to give her room.

"Nothing in the Universal Coverage Manual grants you the

right to present your case before the actual board members. It states very clearly in Section 2622, Subpart G, that the board may employ such means as it sees fit to deliver prompt and equal service to all clients requesting an assessment and/or review."

Hannah snatched Section 2622 from one of her folders. As she glossed over the pages, she shoved them at Smith who did his best to keep them in order. Not finding what she wanted, Hannah said, "There's nothing in here about a computer."

Katie Stuart grinned. "The board functions according to its mandate, Mrs. Smith, twenty-four hours a day, seven days a week."

"You mean a computer does," corrected Hannah.

"A highly effective and efficient protocol as authorized by the board, the members of which were appointed by the governor in accordance with the Universal Healthcare and Medical Assistance Act."

Smith said, "In other words, it's completely legal."

Hannah glared first at her husband then at Stuart. "I came here to speak to another human being."

"You are," Stuart said pleasantly. "Me."

After a pause to collect her thoughts, Hannah went on. "I applied for a review hearing because some errors have been made along the course of my son's treatment. The emergency room doctor thought it was a leaking valve. Another doctor said he was fine. Hey, we all make mistakes. That's why we have review boards, to fix mistakes. If the first doctor hadn't misdiagnosed Timmy then he would probably already have the pacemaker the last doctor says he absolutely needs. Don't you think it's the Board's job to see to it that Timmy gets his pacemaker implanted as soon as possible?"

"If you'll let me read the rest of the board's opinion, we'll all see that the board has done its job."

"Go ahead," Hannah prompted, flopping back in her chair, defeated.

"It is the opinion of the Southeastern Pennsylvania Directed Outcome Assessment and Review Board that the case before it, number 64744215, has been accurately presented. The actions taken on behalf of the client were well within the parameters and guidelines established for emergency care. Further actions taken on behalf of the client were well within the parameters and guidelines consistent with Cardiac Care Level 3. As such, the board hereby determines that the client has been fairly served by the Universal Coverage System. The client is within his rights to apply for continued care within his designated Health Administration District in accordance with practices established therein. This concludes the board's ruling."

"All that from a bunch of numbers at the bottom of the forms," reflected Hannah.

"You should know," Stuart said, "You entered them yourself."

CHAPTER
TWENTY-THREE

HANNAH HAD EVERY RIGHT TO BE IRATE. She'd just been told that her son was back where he started, waiting for a winning lottery ticket. Smith understood her rage; he shared it. What he didn't appreciate was how quickly she focused it on him.

They weren't ten feet from the building when she slammed her stack of files into his stomach and declared, "This is your fault."

Bobbling the files, he said, "My fault?"

"Yes. You've been holding out on me."

"What are you talking about?"

"You've been handling this on your own without keeping me in the loop. You should have told me there were some problems with the system."

"I did tell you."

"All you said was that you had to wait here for two hours, stand over there for half a day, hold hands with some people. What does that mean?"

"It means the system is screwed up, honey."

"Like we never waited for a doctor's appointment."

"Yeah, we waited to see the actual doctor, but I can't remember that lasting more than an hour or so and then only in rare cases."

Descending the stairs to the subway, Hannah chided him for that remark. "I remember waiting four hours to see my obstetrician."

"She was delivering another baby," Smith countered. "She couldn't be in two places at the same time."

"She could have scheduled her appointments better," Hannah replied.

"Really? These days I wait half a day just to make an appointment that used to take minutes on the phone. I can cut that to an hour or so if I'm willing to bribe the guards at the HAO."

This caught her attention. "Bribe the guards?"

"Yeah. You clip a fifty dollar bill to a slip of paper with your name on it and leave them under a block outside where the guards can find it. Sorry, I took the block away. They replaced it with a piece of stone."

"You took the block away? Why'd you do that?"

"Because I was angry."

"Angry?" Hannah repeated. "Why didn't you call the police or demand to see the chief administrator?"

"I had to be careful. Those guards control the line. They might have blackballed me."

"Not if they were arrested for bribery," Hannah insisted.

Changing tack, Smith said, "You took Timmy to Pittsburgh. Why didn't you tell me about the group diagnosis, or did you think that's the way things should be?"

Turning to face her husband, Hannah said, "Actually, I don't think there's anything wrong with a group diagnosis. It gives patients an instant support group. They don't have to face their disease alone."

"Timmy was sitting in a room with a bunch of people six times his age. An old lady pulled up her shirt in front of the whole room."

"So what? They were in the doctor's office, not out on the street."

Smith had heard enough. "I'm taking Timmy to the *Salvare*," he said.

"Don't make any big plans, Bob," Hannah advised. "You don't have enough gas to get around the corner."

Hannah's answer to the problem was to become advocates. They had to shrug off their complacency and work to improve the system. They succeeded in college; they would succeed now.

"I'm starting a group today," Hannah said as they entered their home.

"What kind of group?"

"A big, loud, organized, and properly led one," she explained. "We're going to put them on notice."

Smith supported her enthusiasm with a smile. "Who, specifically, are you talking about?" he asked.

"The Universal Coverage Director, our congressman, our senators, the president if we have to."

"He's the one we voted for," Smith reminded her. "The only one we ever voted for."

"Exactly. Didn't you say he's going to be at the first shovel ceremony at Central West?"

"Are you saying I should walk up to the President of the United States and ask him to look into Timmy's case? We're talking about one kid, not a huge movement like it was when we were in college."

"We can't be the only ones going through this," countered Hannah.

"Judging by the line at the HAO, I'd say you're right."

"Stop focusing on the lines, Bob. It's the care that matters, the quality of the care."

"Timmy's not getting any care. He's getting a number like he's in line at the deli."

"You're catastrophizing. We were given a defibrillator, one to keep with us at all times. That's something, and he's had cardiac reviews all along the way."

By incompetents, he almost said.

Timmy was not among the many things they argued about over the years. Smith felt Hannah should have spent a little more time with him, but she was less a sports nut than a member of the more cultured class, and he gave her slack in this area. But they were not having a debate about whether the family budget should be spent on a trip to the Baseball Hall of Fame or a weekend of Broadway shows.

"Timmy needs a pacemaker," Smith said finally. "Dr. Cooke says that his heart has been damaged."

"Slightly," Hannah reminded him.

"Dr. Cooke also said another attack could kill Timmy. That's why I want to take him to the *Salvare*," he finished.

A silent moment passed during which Smith realized he made the most dangerous mistake any husband can make. He said exactly what he was thinking instead of not saying anything at all. Hannah pulled up short, turned on her heel, and held out an open hand.

"Give me your keys," she said.

"My truck is out of gas."

"I know that. You have a key to my SUV, too. Let me have it."

He gave it to her, placing it on the kitchen table while she continued her diatribe. She bullied him about exaggerating Timmy's condition. Yes, it was serious, but no, he wasn't on death's door.

"I don't know why you're against the *Salvare*," Smith persisted when she took a break for a glass of water.

"For a moment, let's forget about breaking the law and losing the coverage we're entitled to. Let's look at the big picture."

"Go on."

"*Salvare* is the problem, Bob, not the solution," Hannah said. "That boat represents everything we fought against. Don't you remember those rich doctors who double-billed Medicare? The giant pharmaceutical companies making billions on pills people didn't need? Don't you remember the hospitals that kicked people out in the street because they didn't have insurance? People were dying for lack of money."

He remembered those stories, especially the testimony during congressional hearings that led up to the passage of the Universal Healthcare and Medical Assistance Act. Nonetheless, double billing Medicare ended with the implementation of Universal Coverage, which put doctors on fixed salaries. Pharmaceuticals were produced by government-run labs. As far as he knew, no one was left on the street outside the hospital, although they were directed to a different hospital due to staff shortages. For all of that, there were patients waiting in hallways, meeting in groups with a doctor instead of privately, and Mr. Fetterman was withering away with hard cider to dull the pain. Apparently, there was plenty of funding to pay Dr. Solorzano to convince people that the best thing they could do is accept death and joyfully move on.

Before he and Hannah marched in the streets, before Universal Coverage, before his father died and his stock was worth double what it was now, Mr. Porter got a pacemaker and happily tooled around in his '92 Caprice showing off his scar. Smith never heard him say a word about getting in line for it, or for that matter, bribing someone to jump ahead. That was the old system, the one where the doctors supposedly got rich with their schemes, and where the insurance companies allegedly denied claims. In those days private companies operated hospitals, as did the Catholic Church, charities, and various universities. When he visited his father back then, no one lay in the hallway waiting for a berth in a bay suite or whatever Foster called the room designed for eight.

For all the promises of the new system, there was no firm date for Timmy to get a pacemaker. Did Hannah expect him to sit tight while she ironed out the wrinkles with her action committee?

She made it perfectly clear. "I don't want to give the *Salvare* one dime," she said.

"This isn't about money," Smith scoffed.

"Yes it is," Hannah fired back. "Dr. Jossy is taking advantage of innocent people's tragedy. Look at you; you're the perfect example. You have yourself all worked up about minor delays. You've convinced yourself Timmy is going to die any minute. And what do you do, rush into the arms of a guy who has both hands on your wallet. He preys on people like us. Can't you see that?"

No, he couldn't see that. Rather, he saw Ellen Ledsoe touting a 700-mile round trip as more efficient than one to the next county. He recalled a vision of Olga Buckley, blue icing on her cheek, telling him it was her birthday not his. Then there was a smiling CDS Joan Foster shoving paperwork his way because she didn't want to be overtime on a case from outside her district. Above it all, he heard the words of Dr. Cooke.

"I would trust my own kid with these guys."

It was all Smith needed to make up his mind.

"Have you heard anything I said?" she asked. "Anything?"

"I did," he replied. "Every word."

"Good," a relieved Hannah acknowledged.

From that moment, Smith tuned her out, giving her the opportunity to complete her missive uninterrupted. Universal Coverage needed a few tweaks, she said, like a piece of glitchy software, but it was working fine, providing them with qualified people, Dr. Cooke for one, who correctly diagnosed the problem, and specialists like Foster, who made sure they had what they needed, i.e. the defibrillator.

"I think I'll check that thing out right now," Smith said. It was the only excuse he could think of that would free him from her.

"When you're finished, come get me. I want to see how it works, too," she called after him.

In the garage Smith opened the lid of the defibrillator. Inside he found a series of diagrams without a single word. Naturally, the first step was to turn the unit on and wait for the status light to turn green. Next, one patch was to be placed just below the right clavicle, while the other went on the opposite side of the torso. After attaching these, the operator, which Smith assumed was himself, was to wait while the unit diagnosed the electrical impulses in the heart. Upon determining that a shock was needed, the machine automatically sent a charge through the pads. If no action was required the machine did nothing. The AED really was easy to use. Wait for the green light, attach the pads, and let the thing work its magic. His previous criticism had been unfair.

Smith removed the pads, followed the wires back to the body of the unit, and checked for any defects. He found none. Then he neatly stowed everything back in the case the way he found it and closed the lid.

Back in his office, he overheard Hannah on the phone in the other room. "Hold on," she was saying. "I agree some reforms have to be made."

This is the type of thing she'd done in college, carrying a camera and a notebook into neighborhoods where poverty was the least of the problems. She was smart enough to go with several other similarly minded students for protection. Together they interviewed old ladies and single moms, unemployed dads and homeless guys living under highways. To every story she attached a photo and these pages became the basis for an exposé in *The Philadelphia Inquirer*.

As noble as her efforts had been then, things were different now. His college professors, rally organizers, and political candidates gave them a list of enemies: the insurance and drug companies, fat cat physician groups and do-nothing incumbents bought off with lobbyist cash. Who was the enemy now? There were no over-paid executives because there were no more insurance companies. Drug research was a federal activity. Every healthcare professional was a government contractor. Every hospital, including the soon to be built Central West, was a Universal Coverage facility. Did anyone remember the names of the politicians swept out of office by the movement? Smith didn't. Even if he did, was he going to look them up and tell them things hadn't worked out the way they were supposed to?

Worst of all, who was running for office on a platform of fixing the system? No one. There was no dynamic candidate ready to take on the powers that be the way the President had more than a decade ago. Those in office, like his own six-term Senator Lou Carter, had their sights on the oil companies, what was left of them. Did Hannah expect that, in lieu of the President's attention, Senator Carter was going to grant her an audience to hear about a single kid with a heart problem?

"No chance," Smith said to the empty room.

The situation was no longer an abstract concept to be addressed at the national level. It was their son who needed something, and he needed it right away according to Dr. Cooke. For all his efforts to prevent this exact situation, he was now dead center in the middle of it.

Smith took a moment to check the headlines on his computer. Halfway down the list it said, "Hurricane forms near Puerto Rico."

Looking up, he glimpsed the Exxon/Mobil stock certificate hanging on the wall. The blue of the engraved border drew his eye. 100 shares was typed in the lower right corner. He took the framed memento down and pried open the back. Holding the heavy paper in his hands, he heard his father's voice.

"You can take that to the bank."

Just then his cell phone rang. Thinking that his father was calling him from the grave, Smith gave a nervous laugh and took the call.

"How's Timmy?" Doctor Ben asked.

"Fine," Smith replied after clearing his throat.

"I thought you'd be on your way by now."

"Soon."

"Come outside for a minute."

Rising from his seat, Smith said, "You're here?"

"I am," Ben confirmed. "I have something for you."

Enroute to the door, Smith passed Hannah on the couch.

"You should hear this," she said.

"Let's give it a rest for today," he told her without slowing down.

"You're right. You're right. I'm just excited to be in the game." Then, when her husband reached for the doorknob, she asked, "Where are you going?"

"For some fresh air."

At the end of the driveway, he met Doctor Ben, who held an antique baseball jersey.

"Mr. Fetterman wanted Timmy to have this," Ben said as he turned it around. FETTERMAN was emblazoned above the number 4. "It was his uniform when he played in high school."

"I know," Smith said, "He wore it to Timmy's games."

From the living room window, Hannah saw Smith and Doctor Ben chatting. She made no secret of her contempt for his ideas during his last visit, and she was about to drag her husband away from him. However, Doctor Ben unceremoniously departed. Her husband retreated to the garage with what looked like a rag draped over his shoulder.

Convinced that her husband had not been lured into anything rash or illegal, she settled in at the kitchen table. Picking up the phone, she dialed the next number in her address book.

"Hi, Jill, it's Hannah," she said. "I want to ask you some questions about Universal Coverage."

CHAPTER TWENTY-FOUR

TIMMY GOT ALONG WELL WITH HIS ROOMMATES, especially the old fellow next to him, Mr. Bonner, who was sort of like Mr. Fetterman. Bonner told him about watching Mike Schmidt play for the Phillies. Timmy said he wanted to play the same position as the famous ballplayer.

Bonner was regaling Timmy with a story about the old Veterans Stadium when Smith walked in.

"Dad!"

"Ready to go, champ?"

"Yeah, I can't wait until tomorrow."

"I brought you some clothes," Smith said, placing the satchel on the bed with Mr. Fetterman's jersey.

"Wow!" Timmy gushed, holding up the vintage garment.

"Get dressed," Smith urged. "We're leaving now." He was about to tell Timmy to be careful with the wires that were attached to the ECG machine when he realized there were no wires. The machine was gone, too. Was this CDS Foster's idea of closely monitoring Timmy's condition? For that matter, there wasn't a single piece of medical equipment in sight other than a walker standing in the corner of the room. It was a far cry from the space Hannah occupied after giving birth to Timmy. She had her own television, phone, and a private bathroom. This place was more like an army barracks with an attached latrine, except that a sergeant like his father would have made sure it was much cleaner.

"Ready, dad," Timmy said, popping out of the bathroom wearing jeans and Mr. Fetterman's jersey.

"Good luck with the Phillies," Mr. Bonner put in.

"Thanks," Timmy replied and turned for the door.

Departing the room, Smith recalled the man who had been rolled out with a sheet over his face. Would Timmy's roommate leave the same way? He put the thought out of his mind and headed for the stairwell. Before they descended the first flight, an announcement came from the public address system.

"Visiting hours have ended. All unauthorized persons are required to leave the building. Failure to exit in an orderly and timely fashion may result in suspension of privileges."

Crossing the lobby downstairs, a trio of guards corralled exiting visitors toward the sign-out desk.

"Do we have to wait for all these people?" Timmy asked.

"It won't be long," Smith told him.

"Keep it down!" shouted one of the guards. "This is a hospital in case you haven't noticed."

Reaching for Timmy's hand, Smith touched the I.D. bracelet around his son's wrist. He wished he'd cut it off on the way down the stairs. Even if he'd thought of it, he didn't have so much as a Swiss Army knife to do the job. Like everyone else, he had to pass through the metal detector and surrender anything remotely dangerous. Therefore, he wrapped his hand around both the bracelet and Timmy's wrist.

"Stick close to me," he said as they shuffled forward.

When their turn finally came, Smith surrendered his visitor badge.

"Sign out," the guard ordered.

Smith almost released Timmy to reach for the pen, which was perfectly normal because he was right handed. Doing so would have revealed that Timmy was a patient and not a visitor. Instead, he took the pen in his left hand, scrawling his name in the kind of script he never accepted from his son.

"You a doctor, too?" the guard asked upon seeing the signature.

"My dad's an engineer," Timmy informed the guard.

"Could have fooled me," came the reply. "Keep moving. Keep moving."

Less than ten minutes later, they crossed the Commodore Barry Bridge. Timmy knew this wasn't the way home, but he wasn't concerned. His dad pulled a surprise now and then, like when he bought that new bike. A ride in the truck was a rare treat and he didn't want to jinx it. He was thrilled to be out of the hospital. Mr. Bonner was a nice man, but the room smelled funny, and the two of them were outvoted when it came to watching the Phillies or a stupid reality show.

Unlike his trip to Pittsburgh, which had been mostly on the Pennsylvania Turnpike, Timmy found himself traveling on narrow roads through the New Jersey countryside. He hoped his dad wasn't going to give him a geography test or something because he was completely lost. Peering out the window, he searched for clues.

They came to a cluster of boarded-up houses. His dad hardly slowed down as he rolled through an intersection fronted by a disused church and fire station. Next came a restaurant with weeds two feet tall sprouting from its parking lot.

"What happened here?" Timmy asked.

"Rural beautification," Smith replied. "Some people call it I double-E."

Timmy caught his dad's tone and didn't pursue an explanation. The place gave him a creepy feeling, one strong enough that he dared not catch sight of it in the mirror. He settled back in his seat, keeping his eyes straight ahead.

Sensing that his dad was upset about something, Timmy tried to remember if he'd done anything wrong lately. It wasn't possible because he'd been stuck in the hospital with those old folks. He thought maybe his dad had to talk to those people in that ugly building again. That was kind of his fault. Maybe his dad was sore about having to pay more money to them.

If for no other reason, Timmy wanted to break the silence in the truck. But just as he opened his mouth to speak, he felt a spasm in his chest. It wasn't as bad as a charley horse, more like a foot cramp. Then it went away. He sucked a quick breath when the pressure relented and put his head back.

"You okay?" Smith asked.

"Where are we, dad?" Timmy returned.

"Coming up on Vineland, New Jersey. How do you feel?"

"Vineland. Must be lots of vines there."

"I don't think so," Smith answered with a laugh. He imagined the future when Timmy would be a clever guy who charmed women and outsmarted his friends. Letting out a sigh, he flexed his grip on the steering wheel. An hour to go, he told him. Sixty or so minutes.

"Dad?"

"What's up?"

"I don't feel too good." With that Timmy collapsed across the seat of the truck.

Smith held Timmy against the seat with one hand as he braked hard and veered to the shoulder. With the truck parked, he ran around to the passenger side, unclipped Timmy's seatbelt, and laid him out flat. Reaching under the seat, he grabbed the defibrillator's handle. After opening the case on the floor, he pressed the switch, pulled out the pads, and turned back to Timmy. Mr. Fetterman's jersey covered the critical locations on his torso. Smith yanked the shirt up, bunching it out of the way as best he could. Then he smoothed the pads into place over Timmy's skin.

The light came on and blinked, giving Smith his first opportunity to breathe since pulling off the road. The light continued to blink but nothing else happened. He couldn't remember whether a blinking light meant that no shock was required or that it was evaluating the heart's impulses? Staring at the wordless diagrams on the box, there was no way to tell.

He knew he wasn't supposed to touch Timmy while he was attached to the AED due to the risk of shocking himself. But what if it was broken? What if Timmy's heart had stopped? Should he attempt CPR?

Unable to do nothing, he felt Timmy's neck for a pulse. Finding no beat, he shifted his fingers and pressed a little harder. There it was, a slight undulation beside his throat. His son was still alive.

Smith didn't know what else to do? From his days as a Boy Scout he knew that starting CPR on someone whose heart was functioning could injure them. He shifted focus from Timmy to the AED several times. The light continued to blink, and he perceived the slightest motion of his son's chest. He was breathing.

At last, Timmy opened his eyes.

"Timmy! Timmy! Can you hear me?"

"Don't yell at me, dad."

Seeing his son's tears, Smith cried himself. He leaned in to hug his son then pulled back. The boy needed air.

"I'm getting you help," Smith said. "We have a little way to go."

"I feel like I got hit in the head with a bat."

"You're going to be fine, Timmy. Take some deep breaths."

"Why does mom always say that?"

"Because she loves you," Smith said. "Let me take your pulse." This time he found a slow but steady beat at Timmy's wrist. "Sit tight for a little while."

Ten minutes or two hours might have passed. Smith couldn't be sure, but his son's breathing had improved. Timmy was also fidgeting, a sign that it no longer made any sense to have the AED on. Smith peeled the pads off, neatly stowed them, and closed the box. Sliding it back under the seat, he heard his cell phone chirp.

"Hello?"

"Bob, where the hell are you? The hospital called. Timmy is missing," a breathless Hannah said.

Stepping away from the truck, Smith said calmly, "He's here with me."

"With you?" Hannah yelled. "Where are you? Why isn't Timmy in the hospital?"

"They're not going to do anything for him," Smith replied looking over his shoulder at Timmy sprawled on the seat. "Not in time anyway."

"What are you talking about? They were going to transfer him home! We have to get him another appointment for the pacemaker!"

Thinking of those waiting back in the hospital, Smith said, "The line is too long."

"Oh, so now you're a doctor."

True to her character, Hannah wanted to argue instead of solve the problem.

"Honey, it took them almost two hours to discover Timmy was missing. You think they're in any hurry to advance his treatment? I'm taking Timmy to the *Salvare*."

"Are you crazy! I thought we agreed this afternoon that ..."

Cutting off his wife, Smith said, "They'll be plenty of time to fight those battles after Timmy's taken care of."

"He's my son, too, I forbid ..."

"I'll call you when we get back." With that he disconnected and promptly turned off his phone.

"How are you, champ?"

"A little better. Can I take a nap?"

Glancing at his watch, Smith replied, "Let's talk a few minutes."

"About what?"

"About the Phillies chances at the World Series this year." This was the one subject he knew would keep Timmy alert for the final part of the journey.

He was right. They chatted about batters and pitchers, the chances that the Mets would get ahead and the odds the Orioles would throw a wrench into the works. All the while, Smith drove as fast as he safely could to the Cape May Airport. It took him exactly fifty-one minutes.

"Are we going on a plane?" Timmy wanted to know as they pulled through the open gate.

"A helicopter."

"Cool!"

Small airplanes had left the sky long before rural beautification caught up with the power lines. With fuel rationed, no one would tolerate it used for leisure flying by a select few. But as Smith rolled into a parking place, he saw that the Cape May Airport seemed to be doing rather well. There was a handsome terminal building modeled after a Victorian train station, which was consistent with the historic architecture of the nearby town. Plenty of lights illuminated the outside, including one that shone on a gleaming helicopter parked fifty yards away. Two men in flight suits, presumably the pilots, inspected the craft.

"Let's check in with the agent," Smith said to his son.

Although he was exhausted, Timmy needed no encouragement. He knew his dad was going to surprise him, but that he was going for a helicopter ride was off the charts. He couldn't take his eyes off it until they entered the terminal.

Stepping up to the counter, Smith was greeted by a face he hadn't seen in many years. It was Nadzia, Timmy's last nanny, the one from Poland. She wore a neat uniform emblazoned with *Salvare*'s logo.

Recognizing him immediately, she exclaimed, "Mr. Smith! Timmy!"

Wow! Timmy thought. Dad's amazing. He's taking me for a helicopter ride, and he found Nadzia, too. Timmy had liked her. She taught him to say Polish tongue twisters.

Smith took comfort in seeing Nadzia employed by the *Sal-*

vare. She'd been a smart young lady and a good nanny. When she left his employ to study nursing, he expected her to do well in the field. Here she was, looking the part, dealing with patients scheduled for treatment aboard the ship, among them her former charge, Timmy Smith.

She listened carefully as Smith explained Timmy's case, shaking her head at what a shame it was that the boy had this problem.

"There are several people with heart issues making this flight," she said with a glance at a group seated near the windows facing the helicopter. "The cardiologists aboard the *Salvare* are waiting for you. I think you'll be impressed. I was when I did my training with them."

Had this come from anyone else, Smith might have doubted such a declaration, but he trusted Nadzia. She had looked after Timmy before, and she showed the same concern and affection for him now.

"Do you have an approval for treatment outside Universal Coverage system?" Nadzia asked.

"I don't," Smith answered.

"No problem, but I have to read you this disclaimer," Nadzia informed him. "Sorry. It's the law. Here goes ... The patient and attending persons understand that receiving unauthorized treatment aboard *Salvare* is a violation of the Universal Healthcare and Medical Assistance Act and subsequent amendments thereto. Upon returning to United States territory after treatment the patient may be subject to civil penalties for which *Salvare*, her owners, operators, and employees shall not be held liable. By signing below, the patient and attending ..."

"I get it," Smith interrupted.

"Are you sure?"

"I'll take my chances. Let me use your pen."

"Due to the storm," Nadzia said after handing over a ball-point, "you'll be aboard the ship for at least a week until we can reposition."

"A ship? We're going on a ship, too?"

"That's right, Timmy."

"Is mom coming?"

"I don't think so," Smith replied. "She has important things to do. We'll call her when we get back."

Except in the movies and on TV, Timmy had never seen a ship before. Still, he knew there was a guy who stood on top. He was the captain, the one who steered and told everyone else what to do. Maybe he wanted to be the captain of a ship someday instead of a baseball player. He wasn't sure, but he was going to check it out.

ACKNOWLEDGMENTS

The title of this book wrote itself. The rest, however, is another story. Special thanks to Diane and my other early readers. I am grateful to my editor Susan for her insight and Lori for her sharp eyes. Also, I thank Dr. Steve for his medical expertise, Congress for endless hours of inspiration, and my wife Heather for being a 24-7 sounding board. Of course, Mr. Vernon Fletcher's wary countenance is always a reminder to stay on course.

ABOUT THE AUTHOR

Daniel Putkowski lives with his wife and cat in Philadelphia and Aruba. He is a graduate of New York University's Tisch School of the Arts and NYU's Stern School of Business. *Universal Coverage* is his third novel. To learn more, visit **danielputkowski.com**.

Breinigsville, PA USA
13 November 2009

227502BV00001B/2/P